microbiology, immunology, and infectious diseases

The National Medical Series Questions and Answers for Independent Study

microbiology, immunology, and infectious diseases

Gabriel Virella, MD, PhD

Professor
Department of Microbiology and Immunology
Medical University of South Carolina
Charleston, South Carolina

LIPPINCOTT WILLIAMS & WILKINS
A **Wolters Kluwer** Company

Philadelphia • Baltimore • New York • London
Buenos Aires • Hong Kong • Sydney • Tokyo

Editor: Elizabeth A. Nieginski
Editorial Director, Textbooks: Julie Scardiglia
Managing Editor: Darrin Kiessling
Marketing Manager: Jennifer Conrad
Development Editors: Emilie Linkins
Designer: Karen Klinedinst

351 West Camden Street
Baltimore, Maryland 21201-2436 USA

227 East Washington Square
Philadelphia, PA 19106

Printed in the United States of America

9 8 7 6 5 4 3 2 1

Library of Cataloging-in-Publication Data.

Virella, Gabriel, 1943–
    Microbiology, immunology, and infectious diseases / Gabriel Virella. — 1st ed.
        p.   cm. — (NMS Q&A)
    ISBN 0-683-30448-8
    1. Microbiology—Examinations, questions, etc.   2. Medical microbiology—
Examinations, questions, etc.   3. Virology—Examinations, questions, etc.
    4. Communicable diseases—Examinations, questions, etc.   I. Title.   II. Series.
    [DNLM: 1. Microbiology examination questions.   2. Immunity examination
questions.   3. Immunologic Diseases examination questions.   4. Communicable
Diseases examination questions.   QW 18.2 V814m   1999]
    QR61.5.V56   1999
    616′.01′076—dc21
    DNLM/DLC
    for Library of Congress   98-50555
                                                                                                  CIP

To purchase additional copies of this book, call our customer service department at **(800) 638-3030** or fax orders to **(301) 824-7390**. International customers should call **(301) 714-2324**.

99 00 01 02 03
1 2 3 4 5 6 7 8 9 10

Contents

Figure Credits

Chapter 1
The Figure in Question 29 has been reprinted with permission from Virella G: *Introduction to Medical Immunology, 4th edition*. New York, Marcel Dekker, 1998, p. 562.

Chapter 2
The Figure in Question 2 has been reprinted with permission from Freundlich IM, Bragg DGA : *Radiologic Approach to Diseases of the Chest, 2nd edition*. Baltimore, Williams & Wilkins, 1997. p. 441.

Chapter 4
The Figures in Questions 1, 3, 13, 15, and 19 have been reprinted with permission from Koneman EW, Allen SD, Dowell WR, Jr., and Sommers HM: *Color Atlas and Textbook of Diagnostic Microbiology, 2nd edition*. Philadelphia, J.B. Lippincott Company, 1983, Color Plate 20–1, Frame K; and Color Plate 20–2, Frames B&K; Color Plate 20–3, Frame G; Color Plate 20–5, Frames C&D

The Figure in Question 8 has been reprinted with permission from Powderly WG: *Fungal Infections: Diagnosis and Management in Patients with HIV Disease*. Golden, CO, Healthcare Communications Group, 1997. p. 8

The Figures in Questions 17, 49, and 50 have been reprinted with permission from Beneke ES, Rippon JW, and Rogers AL: *Human Mycoses*. Kalamazoo, MI, Pharmacia & UpJohn, 1988. pp. 64, 68–69.

The Figure in Question 22 has been reprinted with permission from Freundlich IM, Bragg DGA : *Radiologic Approach to Diseases of the Chest, 2nd edition*. Baltimore, Williams & Wilkins, 1997. p. 725.

Chapter 5
The Figures in Questions 1, 12, 13, 14, 15, 24, and 25 have been reprinted with permission from Peterson PK and Dahl MV: *Dermatologic Manifestations of Infectious Disease*. Kalamazoo, MI, Pharmacia & Upjohn, 1987. pp. 11, 17, 61, 64, 67, 69, and 71.

The Figure in Question 4 has been reprinted with permission from Koneman EW, Allen SD, Dowell WR, Jr., and Sommers HM: *Color Atlas and Textbook of Diagnostic Microbiology, 2nd edition*. Philadelphia, J.B. Lippincott Company, 1983, Color Plate 7–2, frame B.

The Figure in Questions 6 and 8 have been reprinted with permission from Tenover FC, and Hirschman JV: *Interpretation of Gram Stains and Other Common Microbiologic Slide Preparations*. Kalamazoo, MI, Pharmacia & Upjohn, 1990. p. 14.

The Figure in Question 17 has been reprinted with permission from Stringfellow DA: *Virology*. Kalamazoo, MI, Pharmacia & Upjohn, 1988. p. 56.

The Figures in Questions 19 and 23 are from Koneman EW, Allen SD, Janda WM, Schreckenberger PC, and Winn, Jr., WC: *Color Atlas and Textbook of Diagnostic Microbiology, 5th edition*. Philadelphia, Lippincott-Raven Publishers, 1997. Color plate 20–5 and 20–6.

The Figure in Question 21 has been reprinted with permission from Powderly WG: *Fungal Infections: Diagnosis and Management in Patients with HIV Disease*. Golden, CO, Healthcare Communications Group, 1997. p. 8.

The Figure in Question 23 has been reprinted with permission from Koneman EW, Allen SD, Dowell WR, Jr., and Sommers HM: *Color Atlas and Textbook of Diagnostic Microbiology, 2nd edition*. Philadelphia, J.B. Lippincott Company, 1983, Color Plate 20–6, Frame C.

The Figure in Question 40 has been reprinted with permission from Freundlich IM, Bragg DGA : *Radiologic Approach to Diseases of the Chest, 2nd edition*. Baltimore, Williams & Wilkins, 1997. p. 725.

Preface

My 20 years of experience teaching microbiology and immunology to medical students have made it abundantly clear to me that one of the key elements of an effective course is a well-designed evaluation tool. It is my belief that only with tests that require data interpretation and intelligent application of knowledge will students be challenged to achieve their highest performance level. Furthermore, I have always thought that the multiple choice format is extremely powerful when properly used, because it provides the basis for truly objective and equitable computer-graded evaluation instruments.

Perhaps luckily for me, others are thinking along the same lines. It is particularly gratifying that Step 1 of the United States Medical Licensing Examination (USMLE) has evolved toward a test that includes a large percentage of what we usually designate as high taxonomy questions, requiring the interpretation of data sets or of simple clinical or experimental scenarios. In this book I have provided a collection of items I have developed over the years, in collaboration with the instructors involved in the courses I direct, which I believe will help medical students in their preparation for USMLE Step 1. These items include a mixture of questions requiring factual recall and questions requiring some degree of reasoning or interpretation. A large section on infectious diseases has been constructed which demonstrates the principle of multidisciplinary questions. The questions in this section include elements from several branches of microbiology as well as immunology, and general knowledge of some other areas may often be implied. This book should be used after students have completed their microbiology and immunology course; some knowledge of pathology and infectious diseases is also beneficial. If students use the book as intended, taking advantage of the perforated answer sheet provided at the back of the book and checking their scores against the answer key found at the end of each test, they will get an adequate assessment of how well they can apply their basic knowledge to clinical situations, and how well they are able to recall important facts and interpret data. These abilities will be expected of them as they move into the 3rd and 4th years of the medical curriculum. Our hope is to be of some help in this transition, and to prepare them for successful completion of USMLE Step 1.

Gabriel Virella

Acknowledgments

The author wishes to acknowledge the encouragement and assistance provided by Elizabeth Nieginski and Emilie Linkins in different stages of the preparation of this book. Dr. Carol Lancaster, of the Office of Education of the Medical University of South Carolina, also deserves credit for having patiently helped the author to perfect his item-writing skills.

TEST **1**

Immunology

Test 1

Immunology

LIST OF COMMON ABBREVIATIONS

ADCC	antibody-dependent cell-mediated cytotoxicity	TH	helper T lymphocytes
CD	clusters of differentiation	HLA	human leukocyte antigen
CR	complement receptor	Ig	immunoglobulin
C	complement	IFN	interferon
DNA	deoxyribonucleic acid	IL	interleukin
dsDNA	double-stranded DNA	MHC	major histocompatibility complex
Fab	fragment, antigen-binding	RNA	ribonucleic acid
GM	IgG allotypes	TcR	T cell receptor
		TNF	tumor necrosis factor

DIRECTIONS: (Items 1–78) Each of the numbered items or incomplete statements in this section is followed by answers or by completions of the statement. Select the ONE lettered answer or completion that is BEST in each case.

1. Low zone tolerance is easier to induce in experimental animals when

 (A) Adult animals are used
 (B) The antigen used to induce tolerance is heavily aggregated
 (C) The experimental animal is pre-treated with cyclosporine
 (D) The tolerogen is injected intradermally
 (E) The tolerogen used is obtained from a phylogenetically distant species

2. Which of the following is a measurable effect of successful hyposensitization by a series of antigen injections?

 (A) Antigen-specific tolerance
 (B) Decreased levels of histamine in the challenged skin
 (C) Generalized immunosuppression
 (D) Increased levels of cAMP in basophils and mast cells
 (E) Reduction of the levels of antigen-specific IgE

3. Which of the following factors is unequivocally related to an increased risk of developing hyperacute rejection of a graft?

 (A) Lack of matching for the A and B loci of the human leukocyte antigen (HLA) system
 (B) Lack of matching of the DR locus of the HLA system
 (C) Previous transfusions
 (D) Receiving a cadaveric organ
 (E) Rejection of a previous transplant

4. A newborn with an HIV-infected mother is found to be antibody-positive at birth. The possibility is considered that this child might not be infected, and that the detected antibody was passively transferred from his mother. Further investigation shows that the antibody is predominantly of the IgG isotype and that its concentration at birth is 50 µg/mL. Given that the minimal concentration of antibody detected by enzymoimmunoassay is 0.001 µg/mL, this child can be expected to remain antibody-positive, even if not infected, at least up to the age of

 (A) 3 months
 (B) 6 months
 (C) 9 months
 (D) 11 months
 (E) 13 months

QUESTIONS 5–7

A previously healthy 6-month-old boy suddenly fell ill with a life-threatening bacterial pneumonia. White blood cell count (WBC) was 5,200/µL (75% neutrophils, 20% lymphocytes). Serum immunoglobulin levels were

IgG: 60 mg/dL
IgA: undetectable
IgM: 5 mg/dL
Isoagglutinins: undetectable
CD3$^+$ lymphocytes in peripheral blood: 1100/µL
CD19$^+$ lymphocytes in peripheral blood: undetectable.

5. The most likely diagnosis in this case is

(A) Common, variable immunodeficiency
(B) IgA deficiency
(C) IL-2 deficiency
(D) Infantile agammaglobulinemia (Bruton's disease)
(E) Major histocompatibility complex (MHC) II deficiency

6. The molecular basis of the immunodeficiency affecting this patient is most likely a deficiency of

(A) Nuclear factor-kappa B (NFκB)
(B) Zeta-associated protein (ZAP) tyrosine kinase
(C) IL-2 release by activated T cells
(D) Bruton's tyrosine kinase (BtK)
(E) MHC-II molecule expression

7. Which of the following should remain normal in this patient?

(A) Cellularity in the paracortical areas of the lymph nodes
(B) Differentiation of germinal centers in the lymph nodes
(C) Numbers of circulating lymphocytes bearing surface immunoglobulins
(D) Numbers of plasma cells in the bone marrow
(E) Tonsils

8. The role of integrins in the microvasculature is to

(A) Attract lymphocytes to the extravascular compartment in specific tissues
(B) Mediate the adhesion of leukocytes to endothelial cells
(C) Promote cell–cell interaction in the lymphoid tissues
(D) Promote trapping of antigen in the antigen-retaining reticulum
(E) Regulate blood flow in or out of specific areas of the organism

9. A major characteristic of the immune response induced with pneumococcal polysaccharides is

(A) IgG predominance
(B) Long persistence
(C) Lack of helper T cell involvement
(D) Predominant activation of cytotoxic T cells
(E) Vigorous secondary immune responses

10. When equivalent concentrations of Fab fragments purified from a papain digest of a high affinity IgG anti-albumin antibody and albumin are mixed, which of the following should happen as a consequence?

(A) A precipitate will appear
(B) If fresh serum is added to the mixture, complement will be fixed via the classic pathway
(C) No precipitation is seen, even if complete anti-albumin antibodies are added to the mixture later
(D) The epitopes on albumin recognized by the intact antibody will remain unbound

11. A patient injected with horse anti-snake venom serum complains of malaise, muscular and joint pains, and fever 10 days after the injection. Laboratory tests showed normal serum immunoglobulin levels, low serum C4 and C3, and elimination of 2 g/day of albumin in the urine. The most likely cause for this clinical situation is

(A) A congenital complement deficiency
(B) A delayed hypersensitivity reaction to the snake venom
(C) A systemic reaction to snake venom released after the effects of the antitoxin disappeared
(D) Tissue deposition of antigen-antibody complexes made of horse proteins and human immunoglobulins
(E) Tissue deposition of antigen-antibody complexes made of snake venom proteins and horse antibody

12. Which of the following manipulations is likely to inhibit the proliferative burst associated with an allogeneic mixed lymphocyte reaction?

(A) Adding anti-CD8 antibodies to the culture
(B) Adding anti-MHC-I antibodies to the culture
(C) Eliminating all MHC-II positive cells
(D) Eliminating CD25$^+$ cells prior to the culture
(E) Treating one set of lymphocytes with mitomycin

13. Fully mature and immunocompetent Balb/c mice are transplanted with bone marrow from athymic nude mice. Choose from the table below the lettered choice of the most likely combination of results seen in the grafted mice.

NUDE DONOR/BALB C RECIPIENT

	Bone marrow graft	Systemic effects
(A)	Rejected	None
(B)	Rejected	Splenomegaly, diarrhea, wasting
(C)	Accepted	None
(D)	Accepted	Splenomegaly, diarrhea, wasting
(E)	Accepted	Lymphomas, infections

14. A mature, resting B lymphocyte is characterized by the expression of membrane

(A) IgG and IgA
(B) IgG, IgA, and IgE
(C) IgM and IgA
(D) IgM and IgD
(E) IgM and IgG

QUESTIONS 15–16

A previously healthy 6-month-old boy suddenly fell ill with a life-threatening *Pneumocystis carinii* pneumonia. White blood cell count (WBC) was 5,200/μL (35% neutrophils, 60% lymphocytes). Serum immunoglobulin levels were:

IgG: 120 mg/dL
IgA: undetectable
IgM: 1100 mg/dL
isoagglutinin A titer: 16
$CD3^+$ lymphocytes in peripheral blood: 1100/μL
$CD19^+$ lymphocytes in peripheral blood: 80/μL
Mitogenic responses of T lymphocytes to stimulation with passive hemagglutination–inhibition assay (PHA) and monoclonal antibody to CD3 were within normal limits. Pokeweed mitogen (PWM) stimulation of mononuclear cells was followed by the release of 2 μg of $IgM/10^6$ cells at day 7; no IgG was detected.

15. What is the most likely diagnosis in this case?

(A) Chronic granulomatous disease
(B) Common, variable immunodeficiency
(C) Hyper-IgM syndrome
(D) IgA deficiency
(E) Infantile agammaglobulinemia (Bruton's disease)

16. The molecular basis of the immunodeficiency affecting this patient is:

(A) Abnormal differentiation of granulocytes
(B) Deficiency of the zeta-associated protein (ZAP) tyrosine kinase
(C) Deficient release of IL-2 by activated T cells
(D) Lack of Bruton's tyrosine kinase (BtK)
(E) Lack of expression of CD154 (CD40L)

17. Which of the following describes the main advantage of passive immunization over active immunization?

(A) It eliminates the risk of hypersensitivity reactions
(B) It is effective against multiple organisms
(C) It is more cost-effective as a public health measure
(D) It leads to immediate protection
(E) It is equally effective in immunocompetent and immunocompromised individuals

18. Which of the following conditions would most likely benefit from an immunotherapeutic agent able to prevent the activation of TH1 helper T cells?

(A) Anaphylactic shock
(B) Acute rejection of a grafted kidney
(C) Goodpasture's disease
(D) Hemolytic disease of the newborn
(E) Post-streptococcal glomerulonephritis

19. Which of the following genetic factors is believed to be responsible for the progressive increase in antibody affinity during a secondary immune response?

(A) Allelic exclusion
(B) Antigen-directed rearrangements
(C) Clonal restriction
(D) Isotypic switch
(E) Somatic hypermutation

20. Which of the following membrane markers can be utilized to separate mobilized human stem cells from the peripheral circulation?

(A) CD10 (CALLA)
(B) CD19
(C) CD25
(D) CD34
(E) CD40

21. What is the most likely consequence of a cell mutation which inactivates the bcl-2 gene?

(A) Cell cycle arrest
(B) Decreased cytokine synthesis
(C) Decreased expression of Fas ligand (FasL)
(D) Increased susceptibility to apoptosis-inducing signals
(E) Malignant proliferation

22. Which of the following mechanisms is responsible for the protection of normal cells from natural killer (NK) cells?

(A) High levels of baseline expression of bcl-2 in normal cells
(B) Lack of interaction between NK cells and normal cells
(C) Lack of NK cell receptors that are able to recognize self-peptides
(D) NK cell downregulation by low levels of cytokines released by non-stimulated antigen-presenting cells
(E) Recognition of HLA-C/peptide complexes by an NK cell receptor

23. About 1:100 normal individuals fail to develop antibodies after immunization with the measles virus, while responding normally to other antigens. The most likely explanation for the specific lack of response to measles is that:

(A) The accessory cells of those individuals are unable to process viral protein

(B) The B cells lack membrane immunoglobulins able to interact with the dominant epitopes of the major surface antigens of measles virus

(C) The MHC-II proteins expressed on those individual's accessory cells do not accommodate peptides derived from measles virus proteins

(D) The TH0 cells of those individuals fail to differentiate into TH2 helper cells

(E) Those individuals lack a critical gene which determines the ability to respond to the measles virus

24. Lymphocytes obtained from the spleen of an animal infected with *Leishmania major* show increased transcription of mRNA for IL-4 and IL-10. This finding can be interpreted to mean that

(A) An expanded population of cytotoxic T cells specific for *L. major*-infected cells exists in the spleen

(B) IgE antibodies to *Leishmania major* are likely to be increased

(C) IL-12 mRNA is also likely to be overexpressed in the same tissues

(D) Lymphocytes with a TH1 profile are activated during the immune response against the parasite

(E) The ability of infected macrophages to eliminate *L. major* is enhanced

25. Which of the following is a unique characteristic of Class II MHC proteins?

(A) Expression on the membrane of resting T lymphocytes

(B) Inclusion of β_2-microglobulin as one of their constituent chains

(C) Interaction with the CD4 molecule

(D) Limited serological diversity

(E) Presentation of immunogenic peptides to cytotoxic T lymphocytes

26. Which of the following combinations of antibodies would be better suited to be used on an assay for human secretory IgA (sIgA)?

(A) Anti-IgA to capture sIgA, enzyme labeled anti-secretory component (SC) to detect it once captured

(B) Anti-Kappa light chains to capture sIgA, enzyme labeled anti-SC to detect it once captured

(C) Anti-J chain to capture sIgA, enzyme labeled anti-SC to detect it once captured

(D) Anti-SC to capture sIgA, enzyme labeled anti-SC to detect it once captured

(E) Anti-SC to capture sIgA, enzyme labeled anti-IgA1 to detect it once captured

27. Which of the following associations of complement components is responsible for membrane damage resulting in cell lysis?

(A) C3bBb

(B) C4b2a

(C) $C4b2a3b_n$

(D) C4bC3b

(E) C56789

QUESTIONS 28–29

A 59-year-old man has been complaining of weakness, repeated pulmonary infections, and "rheumatic" pains for 2 years. He has been hospitalized because he broke his right humerus falling from a chair. Serum immunoglobulins are:

IgG: 6000 mg/100 mL
IgA: 100 mg/100 mL
IgM: 40 mg/100 mL.

The patient eliminates 2 g of protein and 500 mg of calcium daily in the urine.

28. This disease is most likely caused by:

(A) A malignant proliferation of plasma cells

(B) A T cell malignancy caused by a retrovirus

(C) An autoimmune disease affecting the bones and joints

(D) Dissemination of a chronic lung infection to the bones

(E) Exaggerated loss of calcium in the urine

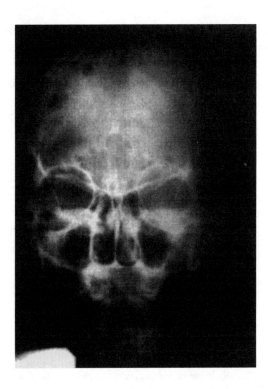

29. A radiograph of the skull of this patient has been reproduced in the figure. The bone lesions seen in that radiograph are most likely due to:

(A) Activation of osteoclasts by IL-6 and macrophage colony-stimulating factor (M-CSF)

(B) Bone erosion by proliferating plasma cells

(C) Collagenase released by activated macrophages

(D) Increased levels of parathyroid hormone

(E) Severe hypocalcemia

30. Which of the following laboratory findings is characteristic of hereditary angioneurotic edema?

(A) High levels of C2 and C4

(B) High levels of C5a

(C) Low levels of C1 inhibitor (INH)

(D) Low levels of C1q

(E) Very high levels of IgE

QUESTIONS 31–32

A 30-year-old man with chronic renal failure received a renal transplant. He received pre- and post-transplant immunosuppression with a combination of cyclosporine A, prednisolone, and azathioprine. He recovered uneventfully for the first 12 days. At day 13 the level of serum creatinine jumped from 1.8 mg/dL to 4.2 mg/dL. A renal biopsy showed heavy peritubular leukocyte infiltrates with lymphocyte predominance.

31. The lymphocytic infiltrate is most likely secondary to

(A) Attraction of cells involved in ADCC against antibody-coated graft cells

(B) Attraction of leukocytes by leukotriene B (LTB) 4 released by activated monocytes

(C) Generation of C5a and C3a from antigen-antibody complexes involving anti-graft antibodies

(D) Release of chemokines by T lymphocytes reacting with the graft

(E) Release of platelet-activating factor (PAF) from activated polymorphonuclearleukocytes (PMN)

32. If the renal biopsy had not revealed any major changes, which one of the following hypotheses should be considered as the cause of the deterioration of this patient's kidney function?

(A) Cyclosporine toxicity

(B) Cytomegalovirus (CMV) infection

(C) Fluid retention

(D) Ischemia

(E) Obstruction of the urinary flow

33. Which of the following is the mechanism of action of cyclosporine A?

(A) Blocks calcineurin activation

(B) Induces lymphocyte apoptosis

(C) Blocks the reaction of nuclear factor of activated T cells (NF-AT) and nuclear factor-kappa B (NFκB) with cytokine promoter sequences

(D) Inhibits the activation of kinases which control the expression of c-myc

(E) Blocks DNA synthesis

34. In an infant with erythroblastosis fetalis, the destruction of Rh positive erythrocytes is caused by

(A) Extravascular hemolysis following C3b-mediated phagocytosis

(B) Extravascular hemolysis following C3d-mediated phagocytosis

(C) Extravascular hemolysis following fragment, crystallizable (Fc)-mediated phagocytosis

(D) Intravascular hemolysis caused by ADCC reaction against antibody-coated red blood cells

(E) Intravascular hemolysis following complement activation by red cell bound antibodies

35. Which one of the following reagents can induce the release of histamine from the mast cells of a ragweed-sensitized individual?

(A) A fragment of ragweed containing one single epitope

(B) An $F(ab')_2$ fragment isolated from an anti-IgE antibody

(C) An Fc fragment isolated from an anti-IgE antibody

(D) Purified IgE anti-ragweed

(E) Purified IgG anti-ragweed

36. Transplantation of which one of the following organs or tissues is most likely to cause a graft-versus-host (GVH) reaction?

(A) Autologous stem cells

(B) Cornea

(C) Kidney

(D) Liver

(E) Skin

37. Which of the following is characteristic of the histopathologic changes seen on a biopsy of a tissue or organ affected by a cell-mediated hypersensitivity reaction?

(A) Edematous infiltrate of the subcutaneous tissues

(B) Periarteriolar deposits of immunoglobulins and complement

(C) Periarteriolar neutrophil infiltrates

(D) Perivascular eosinophil infiltrates

(E) Perivenular mononuclear cell infiltrates

38. What is the most likely cause of progressive weight loss in a patient suffering from a chronic granulomatous infection?

(A) Capillary leak syndrome due to IL-2 release

(B) Increased catabolic rate due to persistent fever

(C) Increased metabolic activity of mononuclear cells activated by interferon-γ

(D) Loss of protein by kidneys damaged as a consequence of immune complex deposition

(E) Negative metabolic balance caused by tumor necrosis factor-α (TNF-α)

39. Which of the following is the most serious complication resulting from the use of monoclonal anti-CD3 antibodies in the treatment of acute kidney graft rejection?

(A) Graft-versus-host (GVH) reaction

(B) Non-Hodgkin's lymphomas

(C) Opportunistic bacterial infections

(D) Purpura associated with serum sickness

(E) Reactivation of infections by herpesviruses

40. Which of the following ligand-receptor interactions plays a major role in the effector stages of CD8-mediated cytotoxicity?

(A) CD2 : CD58 leukocyte function associated antigen (LFA-3)

(B) CD28 : CD80/86

(C) CD4 : MHC-II

(D) CD8 : MHC-I

(E) CD95 (Fas) : Fas ligand

41. The development of antigen-specific T cell anergy is believed to result from:

(A) Deletion of the TcR genes coding for the T cell receptor necessary for recognition of the antigen in question

(B) Lack of association of antigen-derived peptides to MHC molecules

(C) Lack of delivery of co-stimulatory signals to T cells engaged in antigen recognition

(D) Lack of transport of antigen-derived peptides to the endoplasmic reticulum

(E) Release of large concentrations of IL-4 and IL-10 from activated TH2 helper cells

42. Mice from an H2-K-positive strain were immunized with influenza virus. Ten days later, T lymphocytes from animals that survived the infection were mixed with ^{51}Cr-labeled, influenza virus-infected T lymphocytes from H2-D positive mice, and then tritiated thymidine (^{3}H Tdr) is added to the cells. One hour later, cells and medium are harvested, and the ^{51}Cr and ^{3}H Tdr are measured in both. Which of the following outcomes is most likely for this experiment?

(A) ^{51}Cr is released to the supernatant and ^{3}H Tdr is taken up by the mixed lymphocytes

(B) ^{51}Cr remains intracellular and no significant incorporation of ^{3}H Tdr takes place

(C) A significant amount of ^{51}Cr is released into the supernatant

(D) The mixed lymphocytes show significant incorporation of ^{3}H Tdr

43. Which of the following diagrams reflects the fate of a protein antigen injected intravenously into a mouse with severe combined immunodeficiency (SCID)?

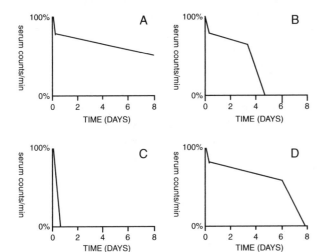

QUESTIONS 44–45

A 36-year-old woman with history of drug abuse and a recent diagnosis of hepatitis C presents with low grade fever, malaise, migratory joint pains affecting predominantly the knees and elbows, and a non-blanching maculopapular rash distributed over her lower extremities and back.

44. The most likely diagnosis for this patient is

   (A) Chronic active hepatitis
   (B) Infectious arthritis
   (C) Post-infectious systemic vasculitis
   (D) Rheumatoid arthritis
   (E) Thrombocytopenic purpura

45. Which of the following test results would support the diagnosis of post-infectious systemic vasculitis secondary to hepatitis C infection?

   (A) Identification of hepatitis C virus in a mixed cryoglobulin
   (B) Liver biopsy compatible with an infectious process
   (C) Positive C1q binding test for circulating immune complexes
   (D) Positive serologies for hepatitis C virus in serum
   (E) Visualization of perivascular deposition of immunoglobulins and complement on a skin biopsy

46. Which of the following is the main risk associated with bone marrow transplant to an infant with severe combined immunodeficiency?

   (A) Development of chimerism
   (B) Incomplete reconstitution of the immune system
   (C) Lack of correction of the defect due to rejection of the graft
   (D) Life-threatening infection
   (E) Uncontrolled proliferation of allo-reactive donor T lymphocytes

47. A deficiency of erythrocyte CR1 receptors is associated with:

   (A) Accumulation of C3dg and C3d in circulating blood
   (B) Capillary leak syndrome
   (C) Hereditary angioneurotic edema
   (D) Increased deposition of antigen-antibody complexes in tissues
   (E) Paroxysmal nocturnal hemoglobinuria (PNH)

48. Which of the following is a major limitation when considering replacement therapy for an IgA deficient patient?

   (A) Existence of IgA in several molecular forms
   (B) Lack of complement-fixing capacity of IgA
   (C) Low concentration in serum of IgA
   (D) Selective transport to secretions of IgA
   (E) Short half-life of IgA

49. The hypervariable genes of the immunoglobulin heavy and light chains undergo somatic mutations during a humoral immune response. As a consequence of these mutations:

   (A) Antibodies of higher affinity for the antigen are synthesized
   (B) The antibody isotype switches from IgM to IgG
   (C) The immunoglobulin genes of the "silent" chromosomes undergo rearrangement
   (D) The repertoire of antibodies reacting with the antigen decreases
   (E) There are changes in the IgG heavy chain (GM) allotype expression

50. Which of the following is the most frequent cause of clinically depressed phagocytic function?

   (A) Cell adherence defects
   (B) Chediak-Higashi syndrome
   (C) Congenital neutropenia
   (D) Chronic granulomatous disease
   (E) Drug-induced neutropenia

51. In an enzymoimmunoassay for tetanus antibodies, tetanus toxoid is adsorbed to a solid phase, then samples containing antibodies are allowed to react with the immobilized antigen. Next, an enzyme-labeled second antibody to human immunoglobulins is added, and last, a substrate is added which develops color in the presence of the enzyme conjugated to the second antibody. The intensity of color after adding the substrate primarily indicates the concentration of

    (A) Specific antibody in the patient's serum
    (B) Antigen adsorbed to the solid phase
    (C) Enzyme-labeled antibody
    (D) Immunoglobulins in the patient's serum
    (E) Substrate

52. Downregulation of the immune response may be caused by glucocorticoids. Which of the following is one of the mechanisms of action responsible for this?

    (A) Downregulation of the synthesis of phospholipase A2
    (B) Increased synthesis of the nuclear factor-kappa B (NFκB) inhibitor protein (IκB)
    (C) Inhibition of the protein kinases controlling entry into cell division cycle
    (D) Reduction of the synthesis and release of prostaglandins
    (E) Upregulation of the release of immunosuppressive cytokines

QUESTIONS 53–54

A 25-year-old white woman seeks medical attention because of progressive weight loss associated with intermittent fever and joint pain predominantly affecting the small distal joints. Physical examination shows an erythematous rash on the malar regions and on the upper part of the anterior side of the thorax, below the neck. Enlarged, non-tender, lymph nodes are felt in the cervical, axillary, and inguinal regions. Laboratory tests showed anemia, reticulocytosis, a positive indirect Coombs test, positive anti-nuclear antibodies, and proteinuria (2 g/24 hr).

53. The proteinuria in this patient is likely to result from:

    (A) Formation of DNA–anti-DNA immune complexes on the glomerular basement membrane
    (B) Inflammation triggered by autoantibodies reactive with the glomerular basement membrane
    (C) Leukocytic infiltration of the renal interstitium
    (D) Precipitation of cryoglobulins made of IgG and rheumatoid factor on the glomerular capillaries
    (E) Tubular damage due to hemoglobin toxicity

54. Which of the following tests would be the most informative in diagnosing this patient's problem?

    (A) Anti-dsDNA
    (B) C1q binding assay for soluble immune complexes
    (C) Cryoglobulin assay
    (D) Lymph node biopsy
    (E) Rheumatoid factor

55. Which of the following monoclonal antibodies could be coupled to magnetic beads to deplete a phytohemagglutin (PHA) -stimulated mononuclear cell culture of activated T lymphocytes?

    (A) CD2
    (B) CD3
    (C) CD4
    (D) CD19
    (E) CD25

56. Which of the following characteristics of tissue-deposited antigen-antibody complexes is most closely related to their potential pathogenicity?

    (A) They are cryoprecipitable
    (B) They contain dsDNA
    (C) They contain IgG1 antibodies
    (D) They contain IgM antibodies
    (E) They contain viral particles

57. Which of the following tests should be used to assess natural killer (NK) cell function?

    (A) Ability to kill target cells incubated with specific antibody
    (B) Co-expression of CD56 and CD25
    (C) Cytotoxic effect on specific transformed cell lines
    (D) Immunostaining with a specific monoclonal antibody for granzymes
    (E) Proliferation in one-way mixed lymphocyte reactions

58. An 8-month old male infant has suffered from repeated bacterial infections since the age of 3 months. After completing his first 3 doses of diphtheria–tetanus–acellular pertussis (DTaP), he is found to have undetectable antibodies to diphtheria and tetanus toxoids. The best course of action to be taken on behalf of this infant is to

    (A) Determine the serum levels of IL-6
    (B) Enumerate the proportion of CD25$^+$/ CD3 lymphocytes
    (C) Measure the concentrations of circulating immunoglobulins
    (D) Enumerate CD3$^+$ lymphocytes in the peripheral blood
    (E) Wait until the first DTaP booster is given and then repeat antibody determinations

59. Antiviral antibodies protect against infections by which of the following mechanisms?

(A) They agglutinate circulating viral particles and prevent their diffusion into tissues

(B) They cause the lysis of viral particles

(C) They induce phagocytosis of the virus

(D) They prevent the penetration or uncoating of viruses into target cells

(E) They sequester the virus in the form of tissue-deposited immune complexes

60. Antitetanus toxoid antibodies protect against tetanus by which of the following mechanisms?

(A) They bind to the antigenic portion of the toxin molecule and inhibit the interaction between the toxin and its receptor

(B) They cause the uptake of *Clostridium tetani* by phagocytic cells before it releases significant amounts of toxin

(C) They create the immunological memory necessary for a rapid response to the toxin released during an infection

(D) They block the toxin's active site

(E) They promote the rapid elimination of *C. tetani* by ADCC

61. Rabbit antisheep red cell antibodies of several different isotypes were isolated and mixed with sheep red cells and guinea pig complement. Five minutes later the amount of free hemoglobin in each tube was measured. Which antibody was most likely added to the tube with maximal amount of free hemoglobin?

(A) IgA

(B) IgE

(C) IgG3

(D) IgG4

(E) IgM

62. In a second experiment, sheep red cells were incubated, in the complete absence of complement, with antibodies of different isotypes (as listed below). After incubation, the sheep red cells were added to a suspension of human monocytes. After a one-hour incubation at 37°C, the monocytes were examined microscopically to determine whether they had ingested the sheep red cells. Which antibody isotype caused the highest degree of red cell ingestion?

(A) IgA

(B) IgE

(C) IgG1

(D) IgG4

(E) IgM

63. A fixed concentration of antibody is mixed with a series of dilutions of the corresponding antigen. After overnight incubation, there was no visible precipitation in any of the mixtures. Which of the following hypotheses would best explain this observation?

(A) The antibody has been cleaved with pepsin

(B) The antibody is of the IgG3 isotype

(C) The antigen has multiple, closely repeated determinants

(D) The antigen has only two determinants

(E) The antigen is monovalent

64. The IgG allotypes G1M3 and G1M17 are true alleles. Because of this, the circulating immunoglobulin G1 of a G1M3,17 individual will

(A) Contain a mixture of G1M3, G1M17, and G1M3,17 molecules

(B) Express both G1M3 and G1M17 in the same molecules

(C) Express either G1M3 or G1M17

(D) Express neither G1M3 or G1M17

(E) Include a mixture of G1M3 molecules and G1M17 molecules

65. A patient who is allergic to ragweed and has hyperactive airways syndrome undergoes ragweed hyposensitization. Which of the following changes is most likely to be associated with clinical improvement?

(A) Progressive increase of the levels of IgG anti-ragweed antibody

(B) Progressive reduction of the levels of IgE anti-ragweed antibody

(C) Replacement of IgE anti-ragweed antibodies by IgG antibodies of the same specificity on the basophil cell membrane

(D) Synthesis of large amounts of IgA1 anti-ragweed antibody

(E) Synthesis of large amounts of IgG4 anti-ragweed antibody

66. The risk of giving birth to a baby with erythroblastosis fetalis is lower for a pregnant woman (gravida 2, para 1) whose blood group is A and who is Rh-negative if the :

(A) Father of both babies is group A, Rh-positive

(B) Father of both babies is group B, Rh-positive

(C) First baby was group A, Rh-positive

(D) First baby was group AB, Rh-positive

(E) First baby was group O, Rh-positive

67. The role of neutrophils in promoting the perpetuation of an inflammatory reaction depends, in part, on their ability to continue promoting the recruitment and activation of polymorphonuclear leukocytes. Which one of the following soluble factors released by neutrophils plays a critical role in this self-perpetuating cycle?

(A) C5a
(B) Elastase
(C) IL-8
(D) Platelet activating factor (PAF)
(E) Regulation on activation, normal T cell expressed and secreted (RANTES)

68. A 28-year-old woman starts feeling dizzy and sweaty 20 minutes after eating seafood. She eventually passes out and is brought to the hospital where she is found to be severely hypotensive. She responds quickly to an intravenous drip of epinephrine. This patient's condition was a direct consequence of the

(A) Activation of basophils with IgE antibodies to seafood antigens
(B) Formation of antigen–antibody complexes in circulation
(C) Ingestion of a potent enterotoxin with the seafood
(D) Release of endotoxin from bacteria ingested with the seafood
(E) Release of mediators by sensitized T cells in the intestinal submucosa

69. A 6-year-old girl who during the last year has had repeated episodes of sinusitis, chronic diarrhea, and middle ear infection with *Streptococcus pneumoniae* and *Haemophilus influenzae* is admitted to the hospital with acute bacterial pneumonia. She had been previously healthy and is within normal age limits for weight and height. Laboratory data at the time of admission show a lymphocyte count slightly below the normal range with 80% CD3$^+$ T cells and 8% CD19$^+$ B cells, decreased absolute number of CD4$^+$ cells, and significantly low levels of all immunoglobulins. HIV serologies are negative. What is the expected result of a repeat of the assay of serum immunoglobulins 3 weeks later?

(A) Increased levels of IgG
(B) Increased levels of IgG, IgM, and IgA
(C) Increased levels of IgM
(D) Increased levels of IgM and IgG
(E) No significant changes in immunoglobulin concentrations

70. A 63-year-old male patient has been admitted for his third episode of pneumococcal pneumonia in the last 6 months. He shows osteolytic lesions in the skull and right femur, a monoclonal IgGk protein, and anemia. What cell population would you expect to find numerically increased in the bone marrow aspirate of this patient?

(A) CD19$^+$ lymphocytes
(B) Erythroblasts
(C) Lymphoblasts
(D) Osteoblasts
(E) Plasma cells

71. A suspension of mononuclear cells from a normal individual is stimulated with interferon-γ. Which of the following pairs of cell markers is likely to be overexpressed by the the cell population which becomes activated?

(A) CD25 (IL-2 receptor) and CD19
(B) CD25 (IL-2 receptor) and MHC-II
(C) CD3 and CD8
(D) CD32 (Fcγ receptor II) and MHC-II
(E) CD56 (N-CAM) and CD16 (FcγRIII)

72. A 6-month-old male infant, small for age, is admitted for evaluation of a possible immune deficiency disease. The child has suffered repeated episodes of pulmonary infection, chronic diarrhea, and chronic thrush; shows a marked decrease of CD3$^+$,CD4$^+$,CD8$^+$ and CD19$^+$ lymphocytes and very low immunoglobulin levels. Skin tests for several antigens (including candidin) are negative. This child is likely to have:

(A) A combined defect of cellular and humoral immunity
(B) A congenital form of agammaglobulinemia
(C) A lack of differentiation of B lymphocytes
(D) A lack of responsiveness to *Candida* antigens
(E) A severe depletion of helper T lymphocytes

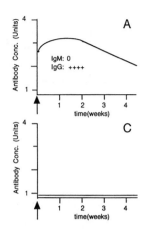
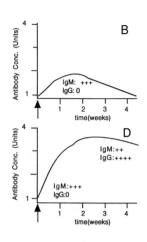

73. The diagram above represents the outcome of four immunization experiments carried out on groups of mice. The arrows represent the time of immunization. The concentrations of antibody were followed for 4 weeks and the results of antibody assay are given in arbitrary units, with 1 representing the lower limit of detection and 4 representing a fourfold increase in antibody concentration. Which of the following hypotheses would best explain the results observed in panel B?

(A) Immunization of a group of animals receiving cyclophosphamide
(B) Immunization with a polysaccharide
(C) Immunization with a polysaccharide–toxoid conjugate
(D) Immunization with a soluble hapten
(E) Immunization with a tolerogenic dose of antigen

74. The serum of a patient with suspected viral encephalitis is sent to the laboratory for a complement fixation test. The patient's serum is first heated at 56°C for 30 minutes, then is adsorbed with washed sheep red cells, and finally mixed with a battery of inactivated equine encephalitis viruses. A dilution of fresh guinea pig serum was added to the serum-virus mixtures. After a 30-minute incubation period, "antibody sensitized" sheep red blood cells were added to the mixture. Fifteen minutes later the tubes were inspected. Frank hemolysis was evident in all, except the one in which the serum was mixed with western equine encephalitis (WEE) virus. What is the meaning of this finding?

(A) The patient had anti-red cell antibodies in circulation
(B) The patient had antibodies to all viruses tested, except the WEE virus
(C) The patient had been exposed to WEE virus
(D) The red cells were able to fix complement
(E) The WEE virus caused red cell lysis in the absence of neutralizing antibodies

75. A mononuclear cell suspension is activated with anti-CD3 + IL-4. Twenty-four hours later, the supernatant of this culture is harvested. Which of the following combinations of cytokines is most likely to be present in the supernatant?

(A) IL-1, IFNγ, IL-12
(B) IL-1, IL-12, TNFα
(C) IL-2, IL-3, GM-CSF
(D) IL-2, IL-3, TNF-β, IFNγ
(E) IL-4, IL-5, IL-10

76. Which one of the following cytokines is responsible for the recruitment of eosinophils to the peribronchial tissues in a patient with chronic bronchial asthma?

(A) IL-1
(B) IL-2
(C) IL-4
(D) IL-5
(E) IL-6
(F) IL-8
(G) IL-10
(H) IL-12
(I) IL-13
(J) IL-15

77. Which one of the following cytokines is responsible for the recruitment of lymphocytes and neutrophils by activated macrophages?

(A) IFN-γ
(B) IL-2
(C) IL-3
(D) IL-4
(E) IL-5
(F) IL-8
(G) IL-10
(H) IL-12
(I) IL-13
(J) IL-15

Directions: (Items 78–80) Each of the numbered items or incomplete statements in this section is negatively phrased, as indicated by a capitalized word such as NOT, LEAST, or EXCEPT. Select the ONE lettered answer or completion that is BEST in each case.

78. The HLA phenotypes of a married couple are:

Father A1,9; Cw1,w2; B5,12, DR1,3

Mother A2,3; Cw1,w5; B8,17; DR2,4

Which of the following phenotypes would definitely **NOT** be possible in an offspring of that couple?

(A) A1,2; Cw1-, B5,17; DR1,2
(B) A2,9; Cw1,w2; B5,8; DR2,3
(C) A2-; Cw1,w2; B5,8; DR1,2
(D) A1,2; Cw1-; B5,8; DR1,4
(E) A3,9; Cw2,w5; B8,12; DR1,4

79. Which one of the following mechanisms is NOT likely to contribute to the immunodepression associated with symptomatic HIV infection?

(A) Death of viral-infected cells
(B) Formation of syncytia involving infected and non-infected CD4$^+$ T lymphocytes
(C) Hyperactivity of CD8$^+$ T cells
(D) Immunological elimination of HIV-infected T lymphocytes
(E) Release of soluble glycoprotein (gp) 120 from infected cells

80. A 32-year-old man is diagnosed with pulmonary tuberculosis and has negative skin tests to coccidioidin, candidin, and tetanus toxoid. Which of the following conclusions is **LEAST** relevant in this patient?

(A) Further evaluation of this patient's cell-mediated immunity should be considered
(B) HIV serologies should be obtained
(C) The patient may be in a state of anergy associated with active tuberculosis
(D) The patient may have generalized deficiency of his cellular immunity
(E) The patient needs to be vaccinated against tetanus

ANSWER KEY

1. C	17. D	33. A	49. A	65. B
2. E	18. B	34. C	50. E	66. D
3. E	19. E	35. B	51. A	67. D
4. D	20. D	36. D	52. B	68. A
5. D	21. D	37. E	53. A	69. E
6. D	22. E	38. E	54. A	70. E
7. A	23. C	39. B	55. E	71. D
8. B	24. B	40. E	56. C	72. A
9. C	25. C	41. C	57. C	73. B
10. C	26. A	42. B	58. C	74. C
11. D	27. E	43. A	59. D	75. E
12. C	28. A	44. C	60. A	76. D
13. A	29. A	45. A	61. E	77. F
14. D	30. C	46. E	62. C	78. C
15. C	31. D	47. D	63. E	79. C
16. E	32. A	48. E	64. E	80. E

ANSWERS AND EXPLANATIONS

Note: Page numbers designated as "IMI 4th Ed" refer to *Introduction to Medical Immunology, 4th Edition,* New York/Basel, Marcel Dekker, 1998. Page numbers designated as "NMS M&ID 3rd Ed" refer to *NMS Microbiology and Infectious Diseases, 3rd Edition,* Baltimore, Williams & Wilkins, 1997. Page numbers indicated as "PAInfDis 4th Ed" refer to *Practical Approach to Infectious Diseases 4th Edition,* Reese RE and Betts RF, Eds., Boston, Little, Brown & Co., 1996.

1. The answer is C. Low zone tolerance is easier to induce when the conditions are exactly opposite to those that would result in the induction of an active immune response. Young, immature, or immunosuppressed animals should be used, and the tolerogen should be a substance obtained from a closely related species, injected in small quantities and aggregate-free, and the route of administration (i.e., the intravenous route) is one known not to result in strong immune responses. Pretreatment with cyclosporine, a very potent immunosuppressant which blocks the early stages of the immune response, similarly favors the induction of tolerance. The mechanism of action of cyclosporine involves the inhibition of a key enzyme, calcineurin, which is involved in the intracellular signaling pathway triggered by the occupancy of T cell receptors. (IMI 4th Ed., p. 337, 500)

2. The answer is E. Hyposensitization does not result in tolerance, but rather in modulation of an ongoing immune response. Successful hyposensitization is associated with reduction of the levels of IgE antibodies and an increase in the levels of antibodies of other isotypes, particularly IgG. This effect is induced by injection of small doses of allergen, and is specific for the allergen in question. The immune responses to other antigens are not affected. As a secondary effect, the local response to a challenge may be decreased, but that is not a measurable effect. Similarly, the determination of intracellular cAMP levels, which theoretically could be informative, is not feasible for clinical applications. (IMI 4th Ed., p. 446)

3. The answer is E. Hyperacute rejection is mediated by preformed antibodies. Only the rejection of a previous transplant can be unequivocally related to hyperacute rejection of a graft. Poor matching (with either a cadaveric organ or an organ of a living relative) can be associated with rejection, but not with instantaneous induction of antibody formation. Multiple pre-transplant transfusions may actually result in prolonged graft survival, by a mechanism that has never been fully elucidated. (IMI 4th Ed., p. 525 & fllw.)

4. The answer is D. The initial concentration of antibody and its predominant isotype (IgG) can be used to calculate the age at which the infant will no longer be antibody-positive. There will be 16 half-lives of 21 days that will elapse before the concentration of antibody drops below the limit of detection. The number 16 should be multiplied by the number of days in the half-life (21) and the product should be divided by 30 (to represent the number of days in a month). The final result is 11.2 months. (IMI 4th Ed., p. 95)

5. The answer is D. Bacterial infections in a male infant with low immunoglobulin levels and undetectable B cells (which carry the CD19 marker) fulfill the diagnostic criteria of infantile agammaglobulinemia. In cases of common variable immunodeficiency, the B cell count (CD19+ cells) is normal to elevated, and the symptoms are often of late onset. IgA deficiency is ruled out by the fact that there is a generalized depression of all immunoglobulins, and is usually asymptomatic. The diagnosis of MHC-II deficiency and IL-2 deficiency require additional tests, and are not very likely in the clinical context presented. (IMI 4th Ed., p. 582 & fllw.)

6. The answer is D. Bruton's tyrosine kinase (BtK) (named in honor of Dr. Ogden C. Bruton who first described infantile agammaglobulinemia) is a protein kinase critical for B cell activation and also believed to play an important role in B cell differentiation. Deficiency of BtK is the genetic deficiency most consistently detected in these patients, and the gene in question is located on the X chromosome. Zeta-associated protein (ZAP) kinase is a key protein kinase in T cell activation and must also play a key role in T cell differentiation. Its absence is usually associated with severe combined immunodeficiency. The remaining distractors [nuclear factor-kappa B (NFκB), IL-2 release by activated T cells, and MHC-II molecule expression] have not been implied in the pathogenesis of any form of primary humoral immunodeficiency. (IMI 4th Ed., p. 584, 591)

7. The answer is A. Patients with infantile agammaglobulinemia have severe depletion of B cells and plasma cells, which is reflected in all the cell-dependent territories, including germinal centers, bone marrow and tonsils. The case description had already noted that peripheral blood B lymphocytes (CD19$^+$ lymphocytes) were undetectable. In contrast, T cells and their territories (such as the paracortical areas of the lymph nodes) are normal. (IMI 4th Ed., p. 16–22, 584)

8. The answer is B. Integrins, such as intercellular adhesion molecule-1 (ICAM-1) and vascular cell adhesion molecule (VCAM) mediate the adhesion of lymphocytes to endothelial cells. Usually the expression of integrins is up-regulated by soluble factors released by T cells participating in an immune or inflammatory response, as a way to recruit additional leukocytes to an area where they are needed. The attraction of leukocytes, however, is mediated by soluble factors: chemotactic factors (e.g., C5a) and a variety of chemokines released by macrophages and T cells. Cell-cell interaction in lymphoid tissues is mediated by other sets of membrane molecules, and antigen trapping is mediated by immunoglobulin and complement receptors. (IMI 4th Ed., p. 27, 147, 198)

9. The answer is C. Pneumococcal polysaccharides are T-independent antigens. They activate B cells by cross-linking membrane immunoglobulins reacting with one of the repeating sugars in the polysaccharide molecule. The resulting immune response is short-lived, memory is poor, and the antibodies made in response to polysaccharides are predominantly of the IgM isotype. The inability of polysaccharides to activate T cells extends to the cytotoxic population, and it is probably a consequence of the lack of interaction with MHC molecules, essential for presentation to T cells. (IMI 4th Ed., p. 54)

10. The answer is C. The Fab fragment obtained by papain digestion of an IgG molecule, is constituted by a whole light chain and the N-terminal half of the heavy chains, including the variable domains of both chains. Hence, a Fab fragment contains the antigen binding site and is monovalent. So when an antigen is mixed with Fab fragments of a specific antibody to that antigen, the Fab fragments will bind to the relevant epitopes, but cannot cross-link antigen molecules, so there is no visible precipitation. However, if complete antibody is added to the antigen-Fab mixture, the epitopes will already be blocked by the Fab fragments and precipitation still will not occur. On the other hand, Fab fragments lack the complement binding sequences, located on CH2 and CH3. (IMI 4th Ed., p. 76 and fllw.)

11. The answer is D. This is a classic scenario of serum sickness. The injection of horse serum proteins elicits antibody formation, because of the heterologous nature of the injected proteins. This takes about 7–8 days, and at that time, antigen-antibody complexes are formed and

trapped in different tissues where they activate complement (hence the low C3 and C4 levels) and cause inflammation, leading to the symptoms described in this case. The snake venom has been fully inactivated at the time and the amount of snake venom protein-horse antibody complexes that may have formed immediately after injection is insufficient to cause clinical symptoms. The term "delayed hypersensitivity" is reserved for cell-mediated reactions that take place 48–72 hours after antigen exposure, such as in cases of skin testing with purified protein derivative (PPD) or graft rejection. (IMI 4th Ed., p. 417 & fllw., 475 & fllw.)

12. The answer is C. The initial stages of a mixed lymphocyte reaction require the stimulation of CD4 helper T lymphocytes recognizing allogeneic peptides presented by nonpolymorphic MHC-II molecules. Thus, elimination of all MHC-II+ cells will prevent the reaction. Inactivating one set of lymphocytes will result in a one-way reaction; but a proliferative burst will take place involving the untreated cells. Adding anti-CD8 antibodies or anti-MHC-I antibodies would eliminate cells not involved in the initial proliferative burst. Eliminating CD25$^+$ prior to the culture would only eliminate previously activated cells. (IMI 4th Ed., p. 207, 309–310)

13. The answer is A. As stated, Balb/c mice are immunologically competent and will reject an allogeneic graft. The grafted bone marrow, coming from athymic nude mice, will be lacking T cells and would not mount a graft-versus-host (GVH) response (characterized by splenomegaly, diarrhea, and wasting) even if the graft was accepted by the recipient. Lymphomas and infections would be expected if the recipient animals were immunosuppressed, but that has not been indicated in the question. (IMI 4th Ed., p. 505–6, 528–9)

14. The answer is D. IgM and IgD are typically expressed on the membrane of a mature resting B lymphocyte. Only after immunological activation are other immunoglobulin isotypes (IgG, IgA, and IgE) expressed on the cell membrane. (IMI 4th Ed., p. 167–9)

15. The answer is C. The clinical scenario includes an opportunistic infection (*Pneumocystis carinii* pneumonia) in a patient with a very high level of IgM and low levels of IgG and IgA, and no obvious quantitative abnormalities in his lymphocyte subpopulations. In addition, in vitro stimulation of B lymphocytes with pokeweed mitogen (PWM), a T-dependent B cell mitogen, induces IgM synthesis but no IgG is detected. The sum of all these elements strongly suggests a diagnosis of hyper-IgM syndrome. None of the other choices fit into the combination of clinical symptoms and laboratory data provided. (IMI, 4th Ed. p. 285, 305, 587)

16. The answer is E. The interaction between CD40 and its ligand (CD40L, or CD154) is believed to play an essential role in the induction of the IgM-IgG switch. Patients with the hyper-IgM syndrome do not express CD40L on their helper T cells. Granulocytes are not affected in this disease and the other defects are associated with different immunodeficiency diseases. (IMI 4th Ed., p. 171, 206, 587)

17. The answer is D. Active immunization is the most cost-effective method for prevention of any infectious diseases in the population. The main advantage of passive immunization over active immunization lies in the fact that passive immunization leads to immediate protection. It is not certain that all lots of hyperimmune gammaglobulin are equally protective against all types of infectious agents. Choice E (is equally effective in immunocompetent and immunocompromised individuals) is not completely true: depending on the type of immune deficiency in question, passive administration of antibody may not be effective at all (e.g., if a patient has a defect affecting phagocytes, passive administration of antibodies may be of limited effect). Choice A (eliminates risk of hypersensitivity reactions) is incorrect because the administration of gammaglobulin can actually induce hypersensitivity reactions if the patient manages to recognize non-self allotypes in the administered gammaglobulin. (IMI 4th Ed., p.581 & fllw., NMS 3rd Ed., p. 83)

18. The answer is B. The TH1 population is critical for cell-mediated immunity processes (e.g., acute graft rejection) that involve activated macrophages and cytotoxic T cells as effector cells. Therefore, if a specific antibody targeting TH1 cells was produced, its application to prevent acute graft rejection would be obvious. The other pathological conditions listed as possible answers (anaphylactic shock, Goodpasture's disease, hemolytic disease of the newborn, and post-streptococcal glomerulonephritis) are predominantly mediated by antibodies, and the differentiation of antibody-producing plasma cells depends on TH2 cells. (IMI 4th Ed., p. 68, 417 & fllw., 520–1)

19. The answer is E. Somatic mutation is activated during periods of intense cell replication, such as a secondary immune response. Those mutant clones with membrane immunoglobulins of higher affinity have an edge when it comes to interacting with the antigen and tend to be preferentially stimulated. As a consequence, the average affinity of the antibody population increases progressively during the secondary immune response. The antigen has no known effect other than binding preferentially those clones whose membrane immunoglobulin has a higher affinity. Clonal restriction is a general characteristic of the immune response, and by itself it could not account for a progressive increase in antibody affinity. The isotypic switch may play a minor part in the increase in antibody affinity, but it would not have any effect once the antibody isotype has switched to IgG. Allelic exclusion has no effect on antibody affinity, but simply reflects that the rearrangement of immunoglobulin-coding genes takes place on a single chromosome, and the other remains silent. (IMI 4th Ed., p. 58, 110–11, 114, 224).

20. The answer is D. CD34 is a marker that allows selection of stem cells from the peripheral blood, the basis for autologous stem cell grafting, a procedure which is becoming more and more popular in the treatment of hematopoietic malignancies. CD10 is a marker of leukemic cells and can be used to "purge" them from autologous bone marrow. CD19 is a mature B cell marker. CD25 is a marker associated with the IL-2 receptor, upregulated in activated lymphocytes. CD40 is expressed by B cells and its interaction with CD154 (CD40 ligand), expressed by activated helper T cells, delivers an important differentiation signal to the B cell. (IMI 4th Ed., p. 168, 171, 182–3, 193, 206, 564, 571).

21. The answer is D. The bcl-2 gene product is one of the negative controls which protects cells against apoptosis-inducing signals. Its inactivation will render cells more susceptible to apoptosis and much less likely to undergo malignant transformation. Bcl-2 has no effect on cell cycle control, on cytokine synthesis, or on the expression of FasL. Malignant proliferation is incorrect because the cells become more susceptible to apoptosis. (IMI 4th Ed., p. 209).

22. The answer is E. Natural killer (NK) cells are believed to receive 2 types of signals: 1) activating signals mediated by the recognition of membrane glycoproteins, which tend to be abnormally expressed in viral-infected cells and malignant cells; and 2) inactivating signals, mediated by the recognition of self-peptides associated with HLA antigens of limited variability (e.g., HLA-C), which tend to be underexpressed in cells susceptible to NK killing. There are no data suggesting that the expression of Bcl-2 is greater in normal cells or that low levels of cytokines downregulate NK cells. NK cells may require high levels of cytokines to be activated, but this does not mean that low levels of cytokines have a downregulating effect. (IMI 4th Ed., p. 210–11).

23. The answer is C. The frequency of low responders to all types of immunizations seems to run at about 1%, and in the vast majority of cases, the individual showing low response to a given vaccine responds normally to all others. The accepted explanation for this type of low response is the lack of MHC-II molecules able to accommodate the immunogenic peptides derived from the immunizing agent. Given the low degree of restriction of MHC-II molecules, the lack of a given molecule could potentially affect several peptides derived from any given immunogen, a scenario that appears more likely than the only other possible alternative, which is lack of the TcR receptors necessary for recognition of all immunogenic peptides derived from that immunogen. (IMI 4th Ed., p. 41–2)

24. The answer is B. *Leishmania* are intracellular pathogens whose elimination requires macrophage activation. Macrophage activation involves the activation of TH1 cells which release interferon-γ, the major macrophage-activating cytokine. Thus, in leishmaniasis TH1 responses are protective and TH2 responses are not. IL-4 and IL-10 are TH2 cytokines that promote the expansion of the TH2 cell population (IL-4), and promote the differentiation of B cells into antibody-producing plasma cells (IL-4, IL-10), and downregulate TH1 responses (IL-4, IL-10). IL-12 is the cytokine primarily involved in the differentiation of TH1 cells and is released by macrophages and other antigen-presenting cells (APCs). If IL-12 was expressed in large amounts, the predominant response would be downregulation of TH1, TH2 cells, and minimal expression of mRNA for IL-4 and IL-10. (IMI 4th Ed., p. 196–7, 201–2, 246–7)

25. The answer is C. Class II MHC is expressed by antigen-presenting cells but not by resting T cells. The interaction of MHC with CD4 results in the ability of MHC-II$^+$ cells to present immunogenic peptides to CD4$^+$ helper T cells. β_2-microglobulin is a constituent of MHC-I molecules, and MHC-II molecules have been shown to be quite serologically diverse. Immunogenic peptides recognized by classic cytotoxic T lymphocytes (CD8$^+$) are associated with MHC-I molecules. (IMI 4th Ed., p. 33–7, 59–60)

26. The answer is A. Immobilized anti-IgA would capture all IgA in secretions, irrespective of their structure, but would not capture either free secretory component (SC) or IgM with SC. The use of labeled anti-SC would make the assay specific for bound secretory IgA, which has SC associated with it, while serum IgA does not. Using anti-kappa chains or anti-J chain in the first step would result in binding of IgM, which could also have associated SC and the labeled anti-SC antiserum would also react with these forms of IgM. Anti-SC could capture free SC or IgM with associated SC and both would be recognized by labeled anti-SC. Using immobilized anti-SC to capture sIgA and labeled anti-IgA to detect it would be an acceptable alternative, but using anti-IgA1

is not, since that IgA subclass is poorly represented in secretions. (IMI 4th Ed., p. 80, 85–6, 92–5, 277–9)

27. The answer is E. The assembly of the five terminal components of the complement system [C56789, membrane attack complex (MAC)] results in the formation of "holes" in the lipid bilayers of the cell membrane, resulting in lysis of cells with simple membranes such as erythrocytes. All other complement component complexes listed as alternative are involved in different stages of the activation cascade, but play no role as effector molecules. (IMI 4th Ed., p. 144–6)

28. The answer is A. The simultaneous appearance of bone pains, a pathological fracture, marked increased levels of IgG and low levels of the other immunoglobulins in a 59-year-old individual are highly suggestive of multiple myeloma, a plasma cell malignancy. T cell malignancies would not be associated with hypergammaglobulinemia affecting one single isotype; autoimmune disorders are associated with polyclonal increases of immunoglobulins and there is no special incidence of fractures. Dissemination of a chronic lung infection to the bones is not a likely scenario; rather, the increased frequency of lung infections results from a compromise of the immune response (the IgG is produced by malignant plasma cells, unresponsive to stimulation, while the activity of normal plasma cells is depressed, as reflected by the low levels of IgM and IgA). The urinary loss of calcium is secondary to bone reabsorption, characteristic of this disease. (IMI 4th Ed., p. 560–3)

29. The answer is A. The radiograph shows the typical osteolytic lesions of multiple myeloma. Those lesions are caused by activated osteoclasts. It is believed that the proliferating plasma cells release cytokines which activate osteoblasts; these, in turn, release IL-6 which activates osteoclasts. Neoplastic plasma cells by themselves do not have the ability to cause bone erosion, but they contribute to the activation of osteoclasts through the release of macrophage colony-stimulating factor (M-CSF). Activated macrophages are not responsible for bone lesions; the levels of parathyroid hormone are not specifically altered; serum calcium is often elevated. (IMI 4th Ed., p. 557).

30. The answer is C. Hereditary angioneurotic edema is due to a congenital defect of C1 INH. This regulating enzyme controls the activation of C1 and in its absence, C1 activation proceeds uncontrolled and causes massive consumption of C4 and C2, as well as release of large amounts of C2b and perhaps C3a. Those factors, having vasoactive properties, cause vasodilation and edema, which may be life-threatening. Because C3 activation is regulated independently of C1 inhibitor, the exaggerated activation sequence does not affect C5 to C9 and C5a is not generated in exaggerated amounts. C1g levels are normal and IgE is not involved in the pathogenesis of this disease. (IMI 4th Ed., p. 153–4)

31. The answer is D. The scenario is that of an acute graft rejection (probably first set), which is mediated primarily by T lymphocytes. CD4$^+$ T cells are believed to play a major role in such cases of graft rejection by inducing a cellular inflammatory process by releasing chemokines which attract and activate additional lymphocytes, monocytes and granulocytes to the organ. ADCC and complement activation are believed to play a secondary role, if any, in acute graft rejection. The release of leukotriene B (LTB)4 and platelet-activating factor (PAF) from activated phagocytic cells may play a role once the rejection reaction has been initiated, but they are certainly not involved in the early stages. (IMI 4th Ed., p. 520–1)

32. The answer is A. Cyclosporine is nephrotoxic and it is important to distinguish acute rejection, which is associated with heavy mononuclear cell infiltrates, from cyclosporine toxicity, which is not associated with major histological changes at the early stages. In acute rejection, there is need for increasing doses or additional immunosuppressants; in cyclosporine toxicity, the cyclosporine dosage needs to be reduced. Ischemia and cytomegalovirus (CMV) infection would be associated with morphological changes; fluid retention (secondary to large doses of steroids) and obstruction of the urinary flow following surgery should not cause an abrupt elevation of serum creatinine. (IMI 4th Ed., p. 501, p. 520–1)

33. The answer is A. Cyclosporine blocks calcineurin, an enzyme which plays a key role in the activation of a critical nuclear binding protein, nuclear factor of activated T cells (NF-AT). The active form of this protein upregulates the expression of the IL-2 and other interleukin genes, and IL-2 synthesis is critical in the early stages of the T cell response, when TH0 cells undergo the expansion that precedes their differentiation into TH1 helper cells. Other immunosuppressants, such as rapamycin, block the activation of kinases which control the expression of c-myc. Cyclosporine A has no known effects on apoptosis control nor does it have direct effects over nuclear binding proteins. (IMI 4th Ed., p. 500–4)

34. The answer is C. Erythroblastosis fetalis is caused by the transfer of maternal antibodies of the IgG class to the fetus, which then reacts with fetal erythrocytes. The density of epitopes on the red cells is such that the density of red-cell bound IgG antibodies is insufficient to lead to complement activation. Hence, neither intravascular hemolysis nor C3-mediated opsonization takes place. The IgG-coated red cells are taken up by macrophages through their Fc receptors and lysed intracellularly (hence, the term extravascular hemolysis). (IMI 4th Ed., p. 461–3)

35. The answer is B. The release of histamine from mast cells can be triggered in a variety of ways. The most effective is the cross-linking of cell-associated IgE antibodies. Physiologically such cross-linking is a consequence of the binding of an allergen with multiple epitopes to a mast cell or basophil coated with the corresponding IgE antibodies. A monovalent fragment of the allergen is ineffective because it cannot cross-link several IgE molecules. An alternative is to use an anti-IgE antibody or its F(ab')$_2$ fragment (which remains bivalent) to cross-link membrane IgE molecules. This type of reagent has the advantage of not being antigen specific, and therefore can trigger histamine release from any cells with occupied high-affinity IgE receptors. Fc fragments, lacking antigen-binding sites, will not be effective. Adding more anti-ragweed antibodies will not cause mast cell degranulation. (IMI 4th Ed., p. 440–3)

36. The answer is D. Of the listed organs, tissues and cells, the liver is the one most likely to transfer a significant number of lymphoid cells. A graft-versus-host reaction (GVH) results from the grafting of lymphoid cells to an immunocompromised host. Stem cells would certainly fit that role, except when autologous stem cells are used, in which case GVH is avoided. The cornea is virtually acellular, so it is the least likely tissue to cause GVH. The kidney and the skin are also relatively poor in lymphoid cells. (IMI 4th Ed., p. 528–9)

37. The answer is E. Perivenular mononuclear cell infiltrates are the histological hallmark of a cell-mediated hypersensitivity reaction, triggered by T cell activation and release of cytokines which attract and activate additional mononuclear cells to the area. Edematous infiltrates result from the release of vasoactive compounds such as C5a, which are generated as a consequence of antigen-antibody reactions (as when antigen-antibody complexes and complement are deposited around small blood vessel walls). Neutrophilic infiltrates are also seen more often in association with antibody-mediated hypersensitivity reactions and eosinophilic infiltrates are characteristic of type I (IgE-mediated) hypersensitivity reactions. (IMI 4th Ed., p. 417–28)

38. The answer is E. TNFα, also known as cachectin, is released by T cells and activated macrophages, two important protagonists of chronic granulomatous reactions. Among the systemic effects of TNFα the inhibition of lipoprotein lipase is particularly significant from the metabolic point of view, because it induces a negative metabolic balance, clinically expressed as cachexia. Capillary leak would have an opposite effect, due to water retention. The increases in protein or general catabolic rate caused by the other mechanisms are not sufficient to cause significant weight loss. (IMI 4th Ed., p. 428)

39. The answer is B. The use of monoclonal anti-CD3 antibodies in the treatment of acute kidney graft rejection, as well as other forms of immunosuppression, results in an increased incidence of non-Hodgkin's brain lymphomas. This is believed to be probably a consequence of the reactivation of latent Epstein-Barr virus infections, leading to post-transplant lymphoproliferative disorders, which may have malignant behavior. Reactivation of infections by herpesvirus is partially correct, but not as potentially serious; herpetic lesions will usually heal after interrupting or reducing immunosuppressive therapy. Opportunistic infections and purpura are possible, but do not generally represent a life-threatening situation comparable to that of a malignant lymphoma in an immunocompromised individual. Graft-versus-host (GVH) reaction is not seen after a kidney graft. (IMI 4th Ed., p. 524–8)

40. The answer is E. The interaction between Fas (CD95) and its ligand is one of two mechanisms by which cytotoxic T cells cause apoptosis and death of its targets. The interactions involving CD2 : CD58, CD28 : CD80/86, and CD8 : MHC-I play a significant role in the induction stages of a cytotoxic response. The interaction of CD4$^+$ and MHC-II may also play a role in the induction stages of a cytotoxic response (CD4$^+$ cells may help CD8$^+$ cell differentiation), but are not obviously involved in the effector stages of CD8-mediated cytotoxicity. (IMI 4th Ed., p. 207–10)

41. The answer is C. Anergy is a potentially reversible state of antigen-specific non-response, and it is believed to be a consequence of lack of delivery of co-stimulatory signals to T cells engaged in antigen recognition. Lack of delivery occurs when the cells presenting the MHC-II/peptide complex do not express co-stimulatory membrane proteins, either because that expression does not take place or because the presenting cells are not activated and the level of expression of co-stimulatory molecules is too low. Deletion of the TcR genes coding for the T cell receptor necessary for recognition of the antigen in question would result in the total irreversible inability of T cells to respond. Release of large concentrations of IL-4 and IL-10 from activated TH2 helper cells would cause a generalized depression of TH1 cell activity, which would not be characterized by antigenic specificity. (IMI 4th Ed., p. 212–3, 343–4)

42. The answer is B. To answer this question, it is necessary to recognize that differentiated cytotoxic T cells can only kill targets carrying the same MHC-I/peptide combination which they recognized at the time of activation. However, in this experiment, the cytotoxic T cells recognize their own infected cells carrying the H2-K MHC-I molecule modified by a viral peptide, and the putative targets may have presented the same viral peptide, but in association with an H2-D molecule. Therefore, the differentiated cytotoxic T cells would not be able to kill the infected targets and Cr^{51} would remain intracellular. It is likely that the two cell populations, carrying different MHC molecules, would eventually engage in a mixed lymphocyte reaction, and the proliferating cells would incorporate ^{3}H Tdr, but this would only take place after 2–3 days, not after one hour. (IMI 4th Ed., p. 40–1, 63–4, 309–10)

43. The answer is A. A mouse with severe combined immune deficiency (SCID) will be unable to respond to the protein antigen, which will be eventually catabolized like any other endogenous protein, and the phase of accelerated immune elimination (panels B and D) will not be seen. Panel C corresponds to the very rapid elimination of antigen in an animal with pre-formed antibodies, a scenario which cannot be applied to a profoundly immune deficient animal. (IMI 4th Ed., p. 225–6; 591)

44. The answer is C. Patients with hepatitis often develop antigen-antibody complexes which can be trapped in the microvasculature of different organs, leading to post-infectious systemic vasculitis. All the patient's symptoms would fit in this scenario. Chronic active hepatitis would be a possible choice because it can be associated with systemic vasculitis, but choice C better reflects the cause of the symptoms. Hepatitis viruses are not known to infect the joints. Rheumatoid arthritis could be associated with systemic vasculitis, but the patient's symptoms do not support that diagnosis. Infectious arthritis is caused by a variety of infectious agents, but not by hepatitis C. Finally, the absorption of antigen-antibody complexes by platelets can lead to thrombocytopenia, but symptoms are quite different. (IMI 4th Ed., p. 379, 422–5, 490)

45. The answer is A. Mixed cryoglobulins are cold-precipitable immune complexes. The identification of a viral antigen in the cryoprecipitate is the best possible evidence of the role of the viral infection as trigger of the formation of antigen-antibody complexes, which are known to be able to cause systemic vasculitis. All other choices would be somewhat helpful, but not as specific. The fact that the liver appears to be infected would not prove or disprove that the immune response to the virus is the cause of this vasculitis. A positive test for immune complexes is nonspecific, and does not give information about what antigen-antibody systems are involved. The finding of antigen in circulation does not prove that the antigen circulates in association with antibody. Finally, the skin biopsy results showing deposition of immunoglobulins and complement would support the diagnosis of cutaneous vasculitis but do not provide information about the antigen involved in formation of immune complexes. (IMI 4th Ed., p. 484–9; NMS M&ID 3rd Ed., p. 324–31)

46. The answer is E. The attempt to reconstitute the immune system of a child with severe combined immunodeficiency (SCID) with a bone marrow graft implies the grafting of immunocompetent cells in a severely immunocompromised individual, who is by definition unable to reject the graft. No matter how well the donor is matched, there is a high risk of graft-versus-host (GVH) reaction associated with the procedure. Development of chimerism would be a good outcome and incomplete reconstitution of the immune system would be an acceptable outcome. Life-threatening infections are part of SCID, and are not likely to increase in frequency or severity because of the graft. (IMI 4th Ed., p. 528–9, 593)

47. The answer is D. CR1 receptors in red cells play a protective role by absorbing circulating immune complexes and carrying them to the liver and other organs of the reticuloendothelial system, where they are taken up and degraded by macrophages and related cells. In patients with CR1 deficiency, soluble immune complexes persist in circulation for longer periods of time and have an increased opportunity to be deposited in the microvasculature and cause systemic vasculitis. The capillary leak syndrome is usually caused by overproduction of IL-2, hereditary angioneurotic edema is a consequence of C1 inhibitor deficiency, and paroxysmal nocturnal hemoglobinuria (PNH) results from the deficiency of decay accelerating factor PNH. The generation of C3 fragments is actually depressed when CR_1 is deficient, because of the role CR_1 plays in C3 inactivation. (IMI 4th Ed., p. 153–7)

48. The answer is E. The half-life of IgA is 5–6 days, considerably shorter than that of IgG (21 days). IgA-enriched gammaglobulin preparations are not available. Even if this were the case, they would have to be administered about once a week to maintain a level of IgA in the low end of the normal range and the cost would become excessive. Low concentration of IgA in serum is the only other choice that represents a real obstacle to replacement therapy for IgA, since this, associated with the overlap of IgA's charge with that of many other serum globulins, is the principal obstacle that would have to be faced if purification of IgA were to be attempted. All other IgA properties listed do not represent obstacles to replacement therapy. (IMI 4th Ed., p. 95–6)

49. The answer is A. Somatic mutations in the hypervariable regions can only affect the affinity of the antigen-antibody reaction, not the antibody isotype or the IgG heavy chain (GM) allotypes. The affinity for the original antigen can increase or decrease as a consequence of the mutation, and those clones with increased affinity are selected to proliferate. As a consequence, antibody affinity increases. This is the basis of the phenomenon known as affinity maturation, which takes place during the secondary immune response. Mutation of the hypervariable region genes would not affect immunoglobulin isotypic markers or heavy chain allotype markers. Obviously, the repertoire of antibodies should increase. The arrangement of silent chromosomes remains unchanged during affinity maturation. (IMI 4th Ed., p. 110–1, 224)

50. The answer is E. By far, the most common cause of depressed phagocytosis is drug-induced neutropenia. Many drugs can cause this effect, particularly the cycle-specific cytotoxic agents which kill actively dividing cells. All other listed defects of phagocytic function (in cell adherence defects, Chediak-Higashi syndrome, congenital neutropenia, and chronic granulomatous disease) are rare diseases. (IMI 4th Ed., p. 328–9; 498–99; 505)

51. The answer is A. The concentrations of antigen, labeled antibody, and substrate are constant in an enzymoimmunoassay for any type of antibodies. The only variable is the concentration of antibodies added to the immobilized antigen. Under these conditions, the amount of antibody bound to the antigen will be directly proportional to the concentration of antibody in the patient's serum. The concentration of labeled antibody retained by the solid phase is directly proportional to the specific antibody which reacted with the antigen in the first step. The concentration of immunoglobulins in serum is an independent variable, not measured by this type of assay. (IMI 4th Ed., p. 277)

52. The answer is B. Glucocorticoids have both anti-inflammatory and immunosuppressive effects. The anti-inflammatory effects are mediated by downregulation of the synthesis of phospholipase A2, leading to a reduction of the synthesis and release of prostaglandins and other pro-inflammatory mediators, as well as by reduced expression of cell adhesion molecules (CAMs) in endothelial cells. The immunosuppressive effects are mainly due to increased lymphocyte apoptosis and depressed release of cytokines, which is a consequence of several mechanisms, including the excessive synthesis of IkB, which blocks NFkB, a critical nuclear binding protein involved in the regulation of cytokine and cytokine receptor gene expression. The inhibition of the protein kinases controlling entry into cell division cycle is the mechanism of action of another immunosuppressive drug, rapamycin. (IMI 4th Ed., p. 496–505)

53. The answer is A. The case vignette is strongly suggestive of systemic lupus erythematosus (SLE). Proteinuria in SLE is usually a consequence of glomerulonephritis secondary to the formation or deposition of immune complexes involving DNA and anti-DNA antibodies in the renal basement membrane. It is believed that these immune complexes are formed in the kidney as a result of the absorption of free DNA by the collagen-rich basement membrane, followed by reaction with circulating anti-DNA antibodies. Antiglomerular basement membrane antibodies are found in Goodpasture's syndrome, but not in SLE. Interstitial infiltrates can be seen in SLE and other conditions, but are not the cause of protein leakage into the urine. Cryoglobulins do not precipitate in vivo and rheumatoid factor is not often detected in SLE. Finally, the degree of hemolysis seen in autoimmune hemolytic anemia associated with SLE is not sufficient to cause acute tubular damage due to free hemoglobin toxicity. (IMI 4th Ed., p. 383–9; 420–1)

54. The answer is A. Of all the listed tests, anti-dsDNA detection is the only one specific for systemic lupus erythematosus (SLE). All other tests (C1q binding assay for soluble immune complexes, cryoglobulin assay, lymph node biopsy, and rheumatoid factor) may be abnormal in SLE and may help to elucidate the pathogenesis of SLE complications, but they are not specific and therefore, not as informative for diagnosis. (IMI 4th Ed., p. 383–9; 403–5; 484–90)

55. The answer is E. Monoclonal antibodies are used in a variety of techniques to select or deplete cell subpopulations both for experimental and clinical purposes. The key to this question is knowing which one of the listed markers is specifically upregulated in activated T lymphocytes, and that is CD25 (the interleukin-2 receptor). All other markers are expressed equally by resting or activated T cells (CD2, CD3, CD4) or B cells (CD19). (IMI 4th Ed., p. 168, 179–83)

56. The answer is C. The pathogenicity of antigen-antibody complexes basically depends on their ability to activate the complement system and to interact with phagocytic cells via Fc receptors. IgG1 is an immunoglobulin isotype that can both activate the classic pathway of the complement system and interact with Fc receptors of phagocytic cells. IgM can activate complement but is not efficient as an opsonin. All other characteristics (cryoprecipitability, dsDNA and viral particles) have limited relevance for the pathogenic consequences of immune complex deposition. (IMI 4th Ed., p. 97–100; 475–89)

57. The answer is C. Natural killer (NK) cells are functionally defined by their ability to cause the death of susceptible transformed cell lines. The ability to kill target cells incubated with specific antibody defines the ability of cells to participate in ADCC, and although the same population may be involved in natural killing and ADCC, those are two different functions that are assessed independently. The expression of CD56 defines NK cells as a population, but does not give functional information. Granzymes, which participate in one of the pathways leading to cell death, are present both in NK cells and cytotoxic T lymphocytes. NK cells do not proliferate in mixed lymphocyte reactions. (IMI 4th Ed., p. 181–2; 208–12; 302–3; 309–11)

58. The answer is C. The primary immunization with diphtheria–tetanus–acellular pertussis (DTaP) involves the first three doses, given at 2, 4, and 6 months of age. In many children, antibodies to the two toxoids are not detectable until after the first booster is given, at 15–18 months. However, because we know this child has had repeated bacterial infections since 3 months of age, we may suspect that he could be suffering from a humoral immune deficiency. Measurement of serum immunoglobulins could prove or rule out a severe form of humoral immunodeficiency. This is an important step because if the child is agammaglobulinemic, administration of gammaglobulin would be indicated. All other tests (determining the serum levels of IL-6, enumerating the proportion of CD25+/CD3 lymphocytes, enumerating CD3+ lymphocytes in the peripheral blood, and waiting until the first DTaP booster is given and then repeating antibody determinations) would have some interest if this child were shown to be immunodeficient and a detailed investigation of his condition were undertaken. (IMI 4th Ed., p. 181–2; 208–12; 302–3; 309–11)

59. The answer is D. Antiviral antibodies protect by neutralizing the virus (i.e., rendering the viral particle noninfectious). This is believed to be a consequence of steric modifications in the viral outer layers which render the virus unable to penetrate the target cell or to shed its nucleic acid after being engulfed. None of the other choices listed is involved as a mechanism of action in currently used antiviral drugs. (IMI 4th Ed., p. 244; NMS M&ID 3rd Ed., p. 263)

60. The answer is A. Immunization with toxoids induces the synthesis of antibodies which bind to the antigenic portion of the toxin molecule and inhibit the interaction between the toxin and its receptor, thereby neutralizing the toxin. This generic mechanism applies to tetanus: the antibodies elicited by immunization with tetanus toxoid react with tetanospasmin and prevent its binding to its receptors in the CNS. The antibodies to tetanus toxoid have no effect on *Clostridium tetani,* do not react with the active site of the toxin (which is not present in the toxoid), and are not responsible for memory, which is a function of long-lived T cells and B cells rather than of preformed antibody. (IMI 4th Ed., p. 244; NMS M&ID 3rd Ed., p. 121)

61. The answer is E. IgM antibodies, by their polymeric nature, are very effective complement activators. Red cells are very susceptible to complement-mediated lysis. Thus, the addition of anti-red cell antibodies of the IgM isotype in the presence of complement will lead to a greater degree of hemolysis than the addition of antibodies of any other isotype. (IMI 4th Ed., p. 131, 138)

62. The answer is C. For two reasons, IgG1 antibodies are more effective than any of the other isotypes listed as opsonizing antibodies. First, IgG1 is recognized by all Fcγ receptors in phagocytic cells, particularly by the FcγRI of monocytes. Second, IgG1 is an effective complement activator and has the potential of inducing complement-mediated phagocytosis. IgG4 does not share any of these properties and IgM can activate complement but cannot interact with the Fcγ receptors, which are the most effective promoters of phagocytosis of all Fc receptors. IgA and IgF antibodies do not react with Fcγ receptors and are not effective complement activators. (IMI 4th Ed., p. 98–100)

63. The answer is E. The minimal requirements for a precipitation reaction are a bivalent antibody (irrespective of its isotype) and a bivalent antigen, so that in the right proportions, antigen and antibody may cross-link in large agglomerates which become insoluble. Pepsin fragments remain bivalent [(Fab')$_2$] and can form precipitates. IgG3 antibodies are bivalent; they certainly would cross-link any antigen they reacted with. (IMI 4th Ed., p. 78, 127–8)

64. The answer is E. The M true alleles of an heterozygous individual are not expressed at the same time by a single cell (allelic exclusion principle), meaning that any given immunoglobulin molecule carries only one or the other allelic marker. However, allelic exclusion is a random event, and there will be plasma cells producing molecules with the G1M3 allotype, and others producing molecules with the G1M17 allotype; therefore, the circulating IgG of an heterozygous individual will be constituted by a mixture of G1M3 molecules and G1M17 molecules. (IMI 4th Ed., p. 111–5)

65. The answer is B. Successful hyposensitization is associated with a reduction in the levels of IgE antibodies, often associated with an increase in IgG antibodies. In the case of hypersensitivity to insect venoms, circulating

IgG antibody may be protective because the reaction to the venom with IgG antibodies will result in its neutralization and will prevent the binding with membrane-bound IgE antibodies, essential to trigger immediate hypersensitivity reactions. However, in patients with hyperactive airways syndrome, the synthesis of IgG antibodies is irrelevant because this antibody is not transported to the secretions—the only anatomical compartment in which it could neutralize the allergen before it reacts with IgE-coated mast cells in the submucosa. Note that IgG antibodies do not react with the Fcϵ receptor and that the synthesis of secretory IgA antibodies requires mucosal stimulation and would not be induced by routine desensitization by means of subcutaneous injections of allergen. (IMI 4th Ed., p. 99–101, 226–7, 446–7)

66. The answer is D. Sensitization against the Rh blood antigens does not usually occur if the red cells of the baby can be eliminated by maternal antibodies against antigens of the ABO group. All individuals of blood group A have anti-B antibodies, and, therefore, the red cells of the first baby (AB Rh-positive) should have been eliminated by the anti-B antibodies and the mother should not have been sensitized. The other two alternatives (A Rh-positive and O Rh-positive babies) could have sensitized the mother, since she would not have anti-A antibodies and the O group carries no A or B antigens. An Rh-positive father could always transmit the Rh-positive gene to the baby, and since there is no information to determine whether the father or the mother is homozygous or heterozygous (AO or BO), it is impossible to make any predictions about the risk of sensitization based on their blood groups. (IMI 4th Ed., p. 462–4)

67. The answer is D. Platelet activating factor (PAF) is released by activated neutrophils and has a variety of pro-inflammatory effects, such as increasing vascular permeability, upregulating the expression of cell adhesion molecules (the CD11/18 complex) on the neutrophil membrane, promoting their increased adherence to endothelial cells, and activating monocytes and macrophages, leading to the release of cytokines (IL-1 and TNF-α) which upregulate the expression of adhesion molecules on endothelial cells, further enhancing the interactions between endothelial cells and leukocytes, essential for their recruitment to the area of inflammation. C5a is a chemokine which can be involved in the recruitment of neutrophils, but is derived from the activation of the complement system. IL-8 and RANTES are chemokines predominantly released by activated macrophages and T lymphocytes, but not by neutrophils. Elastase is released by neutrophils but has no direct effect on the recruitment or activation of neutrophils (indirectly it could cleave C5, generating C5a, which is both chemotactic for and an activator of neutrophils). (IMI 4th Ed., p. 198–9, 481–3)

68. The answer is A. This is a classic presentation of an anaphylactic reaction triggered by seafood ingestion. Seafood antigens are absorbed, reach the systemic circulation, and diffuse through the organism, reacting with basophils and mast cells sensitized with antibodies from those antigens, the result of a previous, sensitizing, exposure or exposures. The activation of sensitized mast cells results in the release of vasoactive mediators, leading to anaphylactic shock. The formation of circulating immune complexes (IC) could possibly lead to similar consequences if those complexes activated the complement system, but it is a less likely scenario for food anaphylaxis. Food poisoning is not associated with shock developing in a matter of minutes. A mechanism involving massive activation of sensitized T cells is highly unlikely, first because T cells do not recognize antigen which has not been previously processed and is properly presented, a process that requires more than 30 minutes, and second, the mediators released by T cells do not have the same degree of vasoactivity as those released by mast cells and basophils. (IMI 4th Ed., p. 433–6, 443–445, 448; NMS M&ID 3rd Ed., p. 455–463)

69. The answer is E. The clinical presentation and laboratory data are diagnostic of common variable immune deficiency with severe hypogammaglobulinemia, probably secondary to the lack of CD4 helper T cells. In such patients, humoral responses to common pyogenic bacteria are not observed, so it is not likely that any significant changes in immunoglobulin concentration would be observed. (IMI 4th Ed., p. 579–586)

70. The answer is E. The clinical scenario is typical of multiple myeloma: osteolytic lesions, monoclonal gammopathy, increased frequency of bacterial infections, and anemia. The characteristic finding in a bone marrow aspirate of a patient with this disease is the increased number of plasma cells, frequently associated with morphological aberrations. Plasma cells do not express CD19 or any other B cell marker. Lymphoblastic infiltrates are more characteristic of Waldenström's macroglobulinemia. Activated osteoblasts are involved in the pathogenesis of bone destruction, but are not usually seen in a bone marrow aspirate. The anemia of these patients is due to bone marrow depression, and erythroblastosis is not observed. (IMI 4th Ed., p. 553–563)

71. The answer is D. The term "mononuclear cells" designates the mixture of T lymphocytes and monocytes which is obtained from peripheral blood by common separation techniques. In this cell mixture, monocytes are the cells activated by interferon-γ. As such, the expanded population should overexpress monocytic markers, such as CD32 (Fcγ receptor II) and MHC-II. The overexpression of CD25 (IL-2 receptor) and MHC-II would be observed in lymphocytes (T and B), co-expression of CD25 (IL-2 receptor) and CD19 would be seen in activated B lymphocytes, and overexpression of CD56 (N-CAM) and CD16 (FcγRIII) would be associated with NK cell activation. (IMI 4th Ed., pp. 198, 304)

72. The answer is A. The case scenario is typical for severe, combined immune deficiency (SCID), with infections caused by a variety of organisms, chronic diarrhea, lack of growth, low immunoglobulins, and low levels of CD4$^+$ and CD8$^+$ T lymphocytes and B lymphocytes. All other choices are partially correct: agammaglobulinemia could be associated with repeated pulmonary infectious and chronic diarrhea; lack of responsiveness to *Candida albicans* antigens with chronic thrush; severe depletion of the CD4$^+$ cells could be responsible for most of the described abnormalities, but not for decreases of CD8$^+$ T cells and CD19$^+$ B cells; but a combined defect of cellular and humoral immunity is the best descriptive choice for the condition. (IMI 4th Ed., pp. 591–593)

73. The answer is B. A relatively low and short-lived immune response, with predominance of IgM antibodies, is usually seen after immunization of rodents with T-independent antigens, such as polysaccharides. Immunization of animals treated with cyclophosphamide, known to suppress the humoral immune response with great efficiency, should not elicit antibody formation. Immunization with a polysaccharide–toxoid conjugate should elicit a strong immune response; immunization with a soluble hapten should not elicit antibody formation, and the same should be true if the animals received tolerogenic doses of antigen. (IMI 4th Ed., pp. 54–6, 219–22, 230, 336, 498–500)

74. The answer is C. In a complement fixation reaction, the source of complement is fresh guinea pig serum; and if an antigen–antibody reaction has taken place when the patient's serum is mixed with a given antigen, complement will be consumed and when, at a later time, antibody-sensitized red cells are added to the mixture, there is no complement available and the red cells remain intact. Hence, lack of lysis indicates presence of antibody, [i.e., exposure to western equine encephalitis (WEE) virus]. The absorption of the patient's serum with sheep red cells was done to eliminate the possible interference of anti-red cell antibodies; if those have not been eliminated, all red cells should have been lysed. Sensitized red cells are able to fix complement, when available, and are subsequently lysed, but this fact does not explain the lack of lysis in the tube where the red cells were mixed with serum preincubated with inactivated WEE. Finally, some viruses cause red cell agglutination, but not lysis, because viruses do not replicate on circulating red cells. (IMI 4th Ed., pp. 270–2; NMS M&ID 3rd Ed., p. 273)

75. The answer is E. Under the described experimental conditions, TH2 cells are likely to predominate in the stimulated population (IL-4 is the best characterized signal for TH2 cell differentiation). Interleukins 4, 5, 6, 10 and 13 are secreted predominantly or exclusively by TH2 cells, while TH0 and TH1 cells tend to secrete IL-2, interferon-γ and TNFβ. IL-3, GM-CSF and TNFα are secreted both by TH1 and TH2 cells, as well as by activated monocytes/macrophages (TNFα), and mast cells (IL-3) (IMI 4th Ed., pp. 66–69, 196–7, 201)

76. The answer is D. IL-5 is a chemotactic and activating factor released by TH2 lymphocytes, mast cells, basophils, and macrophages. It plays a key role in promoting eosinophilic infiltration in areas where type I hypersensitivity reactions are taking place. None of the other listed interleukins has similar properties. (IMI 4th Ed., pp. 196, 444–45)

77. The answer is F. IL-8 is a chemotactic cytokine released by activated macrophages which has the unique property of recruiting T cells and neutrophils to areas of inflammation. (IMI 4th Ed., pp. 196–8, 246–7)

78. The answer is C. The key to this question is to identify a combination of HLA markers which could NOT re-sult from the couple described. A2-; Cw1,w2; B5,8; DR1,2 is such a combination because the only specificity detected for HLA-A is A2, a maternal specificity. The husband would have provided one of two specificities for that locus, either HLA-A 1 or 9. (IMI 4th Ed., p. 38–9)

79. The answer is C. The depression of the immune system associated with HIV infection is multifactorial. CD4$^+$ T cell death as a consequence of viral replication is possibly the major cause of helper T cell depletion, compounded by syncytia formation, immune elimination of infected T cells, and release of soluble glycoprotein (gp)120, which by blocking CD4 molecules on the membrane of non-infected helper T cells may prevent their proper interaction with antigen-presenting cells. In contrast, activated CD8$^+$ T cells may have an important protective effect, by releasing soluble factors which downregulate HIV replication in CD4$^+$ cells, and by eliminating infected cells before viral replication is completed. (IMI 4th Ed., p. 609–12)

80. The answer is E. The negative skin tests in this patient reveals a state of anergy, rather than the need for immunization. Anergy in this patient could be due to his tuberculosis, a concomitant HIV infection, or any type of deficiency of cell-mediated immunity. Further evaluation would be necessary to better characterize the extent and cause of this patient's state of anergy. (IMI 4th Ed., p. 297–8, 604)

TEST 2

Bacteriology

Test 2

Bacteriology

LIST OF COMMON ABBREVIATIONS

ATP	adenosine triphosphate	ICAM-1	intercellular adhesion molecule-1
CAM	cell adhesion molecule	Ig	immunoglobulin
cAMP	cyclic adenosine monophosphate	IL	interleukin
CSF	cerebrospinal fluid	RNA	ribonucleic acid
DNA	deoxyribonucleic acid	TNF	tumor necrosis factor
Hfr	high-frequency recombinant	WBC	white blood cell
HIV	human immunodeficiency virus		

LIST OF BACTERIA

E. coli	*Escherichia coli*	*N. meningitidis*	*Neisseria meningitidis*
H. influenzae	*Haemophilus influenzae*	*S. pneumoniae*	*Streptococcus pneumoniae*
H. pylori	*Helicobacter pylori*		

DIRECTIONS: (Items 1–75) Each of the numbered items or incomplete statements in this section is followed by answers or by completions of the statement. Select the ONE lettered answer or completion that is BEST in each case.

1. A strain of *E. coli* is isolated with the following properties: it expresses a functional *lac* operon (*lac+*) and can transfer this trait efficiently to *lac*-negative (*lac−*) strains. The *lac−* strains which become *lac+* can transfer this trait to other *lac−* strains. The transfer process is not affected by DNAse added to the medium but is inhibited if the strains are incubated in 2 communicating chambers separated by a 0.4 m filter that excludes bacteria (but not viruses). Under these circumstances, the transfer of the *lac+* trait must involve

  (A) Conjugation involving an F+ plasmid
  (B) Conjugation involving an Hfr strain
  (C) Generalized transduction
  (D) Specialized transduction
  (E) Transformation

2. Which of the following structures are the cellular receptors that allow the attachment of *Vibrio cholerae* to the brush border of the small bowel mucosa?

  (A) Cell membrane gangliosides
  (B) Duffy red cell antigen
  (C) ICAM-1
  (D) Outer membrane proteins
  (E) Sialated Lewis^b antigen

3. The secretion of diphtheria toxin by a lysogenized *Corynebacterium diphtheriae* is controlled by

  (A) A phage repressor protein
  (B) A protease that cleaves the toxin into two moieties
  (C) An iron-dependent *tox* gene repressor protein
  (D) The change from lysogenic to lytic infection
  (E) The levels of antitoxin antibodies

4. A 55-year-old woman treated with clindamycin for *Pseudomonas aeruginosa* pyelonephritis starts to complain of nausea, chills, abdominal discomfort, and diarrhea at the end of a week of antibiotherapy. Her temperature is 39.5°C and colonoscopy reveals membrane-like exudates attached to the colonic mucosa. The pathogenesis of this condition involves overgrowth of

  (A) Antibiotic-resistant *Candida albicans*
  (B) Gram-negative, nonlactose-fermenting rods that produce a potent cytotoxin
  (C) Gram-negative, lactose-fermenting rods that secrete an adenylate cyclase-activating toxin
  (D) Gram-positive rods that secrete potent cytotoxins
  (E) Protease-secreting *Entamoeba histolytica*

5. Which of the following is the common characteristic of plasmid-coded virulence factors?

(A) Enzymatic activity
(B) Expression by a fraction of the isolates of a given species
(C) Inducibility
(D) Protection against immune defense mechanisms
(E) Secretion under conditions of metabolic stress

6. A 6-year-old child presents with a febrile disease associated with an enlarged, tender and hot lymph node in the right axillary region. A scratch scar can be seen on the dorsal aspect of the right hand. The child's mother states that she is not sure how that scar was acquired, but she has two cats and a puppy. This disease is most likely caused by

(A) *Bartonella bacilliformis*
(B) *Bartonella henselae*
(C) *Francisella tularensis*
(D) *Pasteurella multocida*
(E) *Yersinia pestis*

7. What is the best parameter for taxonomic classification of a newly isolated bacterium?

(A) Comparison of 16S RNA sequences
(B) Comparison of G:C pairs
(C) Complete inventory of its phenotypic characteristics
(D) Primary sequence of bacterial DNA
(E) Reactivity with antisera specific for related bacteria

8. A bacteriological examination of a newborn girl with suspected meningitis results in the isolation of a gram-positive pleomorphic rod that grew on sheep agar under increased CO_2 tension and is catalase-positive. The most adequate antibiotic for treating this patient is one that will

(A) Cause misreading of bacterial mRNA
(B) Inactivate DNA-dependent RNA polymerase
(C) Inhibit DNA gyrase
(D) Inhibit peptidoglycan cross-linking
(E) Prevent elongation of bacterial polypeptide chains

9. Which of the following organisms is most likely to be isolated from the CSF of a properly immunized 2-year-old with meningitis?

(A) *E. coli*
(B) Group A *Streptococcus*
(C) Group B *Streptococcus*
(D) *H. influenzae* type B
(E) *N. meningitidis*

10. Of the following infections, which is most likely to be classified as opportunistic?

(A) Brucellosis in the child of a migrant worker
(B) Giardiasis in a nursery staff member
(C) Pelvic inflammatory disease caused by *Chlamydia* in a young, sexually active female
(D) Pulmonary tuberculosis in a young medicine resident
(E) *Salmonella enteritidis* osteomyelitis in a patient with sickle cell anemia

QUESTIONS 11–12

A patient is admitted to the hospital in mid-September with a complaint of 2 days of fever, muscle aches, and severe headache. He tells you that approximately 1 week before while camping in the Blue Ridge mountains in North Carolina, he was bitten by a tick. The only findings on physical examination are a temperature of 103°F and diffuse muscle tenderness. Flexion of the neck is painful.

11. The most important step in this patient's management should be to

(A) Ask for a Weil-Felix test and keep the patient under close observation
(B) Draw CSF and send it for Gram stain and culture
(C) Obtain a muscle biopsy and ask for direct immunofluorescence study for *Rickettsia rickettsii*
(D) Send blood to the microbiology laboratory for cultures and wait for the results
(E) Start therapy with either doxycycline or chloramphenicol

12. The bacterium responsible for this disease is best described as

(A) Acid-fast
(B) Anaerobic
(C) Gram-negative
(D) Obligatory intracellular
(E) Opportunistic

13. A 35-year-old migrant worker is admitted to the hospital with high fever and malaise. He started feeling weak 3 days before; he had a slightly elevated temperature. Because he felt progressively worse and his temperature rose to 103°F, he was taken to the emergency room. The physical examination revealed a tender abdomen and a few rose-colored spots on the trunk. The patient was admitted for further evaluation. He reveals that at least one other worker in his group has been sick with similar symptoms. Which of the following tests do you think would most likely give you a diagnosis?

(A) Biopsy of the skin lesions
(B) Blood cultures
(C) CSF Gram stain and culture
(D) Serological tests for *Brucella*
(E) Serologies for common viruses (measles, rubella)

QUESTIONS 14–15

Mr. and Mrs. Jones returned from a vacation in Cancun, Mexico, 14 days before being brought to the emergency room at 2:00 AM on April 6 by the local rescue squad. Both were suffering from violent diarrhea and vomiting which had begun around midnight. They were given intravenous fluids and discharged the following afternoon.

14. To help make a preliminary diagnosis, ask for

(A) A history of places they had visited while on vacation
(B) A list of food products they may have brought with them from their trip
(C) A list of foods eaten for dinner on April 5
(D) A list of foods eaten while on vacation
(E) A list of friends that accompanied them on vacation

15. This type of gastroenteritis is most likely a consequence of

(A) An allergic reaction to food ingested a few hours earlier
(B) Effacing of the small intestine epithelial villi
(C) Inflammatory infiltration of the mucosa
(D) Release of microbial proteases
(E) Ingestion of a potent exotoxin

16. A sheep farmer has been treated for a febrile disease with flu-like symptoms and progressive debilitation with a variety of antibiotics, including cephalexin, rifampin, ciprofloxacin, and gentamicin. Despite therapy, the patient continues to deteriorate and develops full-blown pneumonia. Which of the following agents should be investigated as a possible cause of this disease?

(A) *Chlamydia psittaci*
(B) *Coxiella burnetii*
(C) *Brucella abortus*
(D) *Bartonella henselae*
(E) *Pasteurella multocida*

17. A bacterium grown in the presence of equal concentrations of glucose and lactose will first utilize glucose. During the period of glucose utilization the *lac* operon is inactive due to

(A) Activation of a catabolite repressor gene
(B) Binding of the repressor protein to the operator region
(C) High levels of cAMP associated with glucose metabolism
(D) Lack of binding of the catabolite activator protein to the *lac* operon promoter
(E) Lack of uptake of lactose

18. A 22-year-old woman developed a urinary tract infection during her honeymoon. When she sought medical advice, she was febrile, complained of dysuria and flank pain, and had cloudy urine that contained granular casts. Urine culture yielded a lactose fermenter, indole-positive, gram-negative bacillus. The ability of this responsible organism to infect the urinary tract is with specific

(A) Exotoxins
(B) K antigens
(C) O antigens
(D) P fimbriae
(E) Plasmids

19. What is the mechanism responsible for the relapsing fever caused by *Borrelia recurrentis*?

(A) Depression of the immune system
(B) Development of antibiotic resistance
(C) Emergence of antigenic mutants
(D) Infection with multiple strains of this organism
(E) Intracellular sequestration of the organism

QUESTIONS 20–22

A 3-year-old girl was taken to her pediatrician's office with several quarter-sized honey-crusted lesions on the legs, characteristic of impetigo.

20. Of the organisms that most frequently cause this type of skin infection in a child, a common property is that they

(A) Are colored red when counter-stained with safranin
(B) Are difficult to grow in conventional bacteriological culture media
(C) Do not grow in anaerobic conditions
(D) Have cell walls with a thick peptidoglycan layer
(E) Have antiphagocytic polysaccharide capsules

21. The choice of an antibiotic to treat this skin infection must take into consideration the

(A) Frequent synthesis of β-lactamases by one of the organisms potentially involved
(B) Lack of effect of antibiotics that inhibit cell wall biosynthesis
(C) Lack of penetration of β-lactams through the cell wall of the most likely causative agents
(D) Need to use 3 or more antibiotics in combination
(E) Poor intestinal absorption of the most effective antibiotics

22. Which of the following is a nonsuppurative sequelae that could develop in this child?

(A) Arthritis
(B) Carditis
(C) Erysipelas
(D) Glomerulonephritis
(E) Toxic shock

23. Radiolabeled leucine, ribose, thymidine, and uridine were added to the culture medium of a bacterial culture sensitive to rifampin, erythromycin, chloramphenicol, and nalidixic acid. Which of the radiolabeled compounds would IMMEDIATELY fail to incorporate into the bacteria after addition of a macrolide antibiotic?

(A) Leucine
(B) Ribose
(C) Thymine
(D) Uracil

24. Of the following bacterial components, which is most likely mutated in a bacterial isolate found to be resistant to ciprofloxacin?

(A) 30S ribosomal unit
(B) 50S ribosomal unit
(C) DNA gyrase
(D) RNA polymerase (β subunit)
(E) Transpeptidase

25. Which of the following properties of bacterial polysaccharide capsules explains their role as virulence factors?

(A) Complement activation by the alternative pathway
(B) Inhibition of the penetration of antibiotics inside the bacterial cells
(C) Inhibition of phagocytosis
(D) Poor immunogenicity
(E) Structural homology with mammalian cell membrane antigens

26. Which of the following steps is currently considered as the most useful to produce a more efficient *S. pneumoniae* vaccine?

(A) Administration by aerosol
(B) Conjugate the bacterial polysaccharides with a protein carrier
(C) Increase the number of strains in the vaccine
(D) Use a more potent adjuvant
(E) Use complete killed bacteria instead of polysaccharides

27. A tetracycline (tet)-sensitive, tryptophan (trp), and histidine (his) auxotroph *E. coli* is mixed in equal proportions with a tet-resistant Hfr prototroph of the same species in medium containing trp, his, and DNAse. After a suitable period of time, the culture is seeded in media containing different combinations of tet, trp, and his. The results of these cultures showed that tet-resistant organisms were prototrophic in 70% of the cases, but of the remaining 30% tet-resistant organisms, 60% required trp for growth and 40% required both trp and his. Which of the following conclusions concerning the three genes involved in this experiment is supported by the data?

(A) All tet-resistant bacteria derived from the original prototrophs
(B) The his gene is closer to the tet-resistance gene than the trp gene
(C) Transmission of genes from prototrophs to auxotrophs involved transformation
(D) The trp and his genes are very closely located
(E) The trp gene is the one closest to the origin of replication (O)

28. Why are nitroimidazoles only effective against anaerobic organisms?

(A) Anaerobic fermentation lowers the pH to optimal values for imidazoles

(B) Catalase and superoxide dismutase inactivate the imidazoles

(C) In the presence of high ATP levels, nitroimidazoles undergo phosphorylative inactivation

(D) Only anaerobes can generate DNA-alkylating metabolites from imidazoles

(E) The imidazoles are quickly oxidized and inactivated by atmospheric oxygen

29. A 65-year-old woman develops profuse watery diarrhea during a flight from Lima, Perú. She is immediately transported to a hospital where she is found to be dehydrated and immediately placed on intravenous fluids. This patient's diarrhea is most likely caused by

(A) Activation of a guanylate cyclase protein by a bacterial exotoxin

(B) Activation of adenyl cyclase by a bacterial exotoxin

(C) Effacing of intestinal villi

(D) Exaggerated intestinal peristalsis

(E) Release of a potent cytotoxin

30. To develop a vaccine, which component or product of *H. pylori* should be the BEST candidate?

(A) Cell wall lipopolysaccharide

(B) IgA protease

(C) Lewis[b] binding adhesin

(D) Urease

(E) Vacuolating cytotoxin A

31. Which one of the following immunizations is recommended to be administered IMMEDIATELY after birth?

(A) Diphtheria-tetanus-pertussis (DTP)

(B) *H. influenzae* type B (HiB)

(C) Hepatitis B

(D) HIV

(E) Polio vaccine

32. A 40-year-old mother of 4 underwent surgery to remove an ovarian cyst. Three days later she was readmitted to the hospital with general complaints of fever (39°C), malaise, anorexia, and flank pain. Her bladder had been catheterized during her first admission and review of her records showed that she had fever 24 hours after surgery. She had been treated with ampicillin. At this time a clean-catch urine specimen was obtained and found to contain pus cells, casts and numerous gram-negative rods. A urine culture yielded colonies of an oxidase-positive bacteria whose colonies have a mucoid aspect and release a green diffusible pigment. The causal agent of this condition is likely to be

(A) *Enterococcus*

(B) *E. coli*

(C) *Klebsiella pneumoniae*

(D) *Proteus mirabilis*

(E) *Pseudomonas aeruginosa*

33. You have isolated an organism that grows in blood agar and forms round, smooth, pale yellow colonies surrounded by a narrow area of hemolysis; ferments mannitol; and is both catalase- and coagulase-positive. You should be concerned about the possibility that this organism may

(A) Be a facultative intracellular bacteria

(B) Be resistant to β-lactam antimicrobials

(C) Cause postinfectious complications, such as glomerulonephritis

(D) Release a potent endotoxin

(E) Release a potent neurotoxin

QUESTIONS 34–35

A 10-year-old boy persuades his father to buy him a freshwater aquarium after receiving straight A's in school. To his father's surprise, he even takes care of the aquarium. A month later he shows his father an ulcerated and indurated nodular lesion in the base of his right thumb. He claims that the lesion developed from a cut he made on that particular spot while cleaning the rocks inside the aquarium.

34. This lesion is likely to be caused by an organism with the following characteristics:

(A) Acid-fast rod, grows best at temperatures below 37°C

(B) Aerobic, gram-positive coccus, easily identified by culture in mannitol-salt agar

(C) Branching, filamentous, partially acid fast

(D) Gram-negative rod, strict aerobe, oxidase-positive, pyocyanin-producer

(E) Gram-negative, curvy rod, grows best in media with high salt concentration

35. This boy would best be treated with

(A) A cephalosporin combined with an aminoglycoside
(B) Doxycycline
(C) Penicillin G
(D) Rifampin, isoniazid, and clarithromycin
(E) Surgical excision

QUESTIONS 36–38

A 73-year-old veteran who has smoked 1–2 packs of cigarettes per day since he was 16 years old is seen at the emergency room with cough, fever (104.2°F) of 4 days' duration and diarrhea for 2 days. His past medical history includes chronic bronchitis for the last 20 years. A chest radiograph shows intensification of the interstitium in both lungs and an ill-defined consolidation area in the lower right lobe. A sputum sample is obtained and microscopic examination shows abundant leukocytes, including polymorphonuclear leukocytes and mononuclear cells. A Gram stain and an acid-fast stain of the sputum are negative.

36. To empirically treat this infection, which of the following antimicrobials should be included?

(A) Doxycycline
(B) Erythromycin
(C) Isoniazid
(D) Metronidazole
(E) Penicillin G

37. A bronchial lavage sample and a transbronchial biopsy sample are obtained and cultures in several media are ordered in an attempt to identify the causative agent of this patient's infection. Which of the following media is the most ineffective for this purpose?

(A) Blood agar
(B) Charcoal-yeast extract with cysteine
(C) Chocolate agar
(D) Lowenstein-Jensen culture medium
(E) Thayer-Martin agar

38. Which of the following diagnostic approaches is preferable as an alternative to the cultures described above?

(A) Blood cultures in blood agar, charcoal-yeast extract with cysteine, and Lowenstein-Jensen culture medium
(B) Detection of microbial antigens in the urine by enzyme immunoassay
(C) Detection of specific antibodies in serum by enzyme immunoassay
(D) Fecal cultures in MacConkey agar and blood agar
(E) Methenamine-silver staining of a cytospin preparation of the bronchoalveolar lavage fluid

QUESTIONS 39–40

A bacteriological examination of the CSF of a 6-year-old girl with suspected meningitis results in the isolation of a gram-negative diplococcus that grew in chocolate agar and is oxidase-positive.

39. Which is the greatest immediate concern in this patient?

(A) Development of a severe form of septic shock
(B) Dissemination of the infection to other organs
(C) Lack of effect of most common antimicrobials
(D) Possible neurologic complications

40. The most adequate antibiotic for treating this patient is one that will

(A) Cause misreading of bacterial mRNA
(B) Inactivate DNA-dependent RNA polymerase
(C) Inhibit the activity of DNA gyrase
(D) Inhibit peptidoglycan cross-linking
(E) Prevent elongation of bacterial polypeptide chains

41. Cultures of 2 neomycin-sensitive strains of *E. coli* are mixed and cultured in the presence of neomycin. After 2 hours the mixture is plated on neomycin-containing agar. A few neomycin-resistant colonies grow. The emergence of these resistant strains most likely resulted from

(A) Conjugation
(B) Penicillin-induced mutation
(C) Spontaneous mutation
(D) Transduction
(E) Transformation

42. The reverse mutation of an auxotrophic strain of *E. coli* with an inactive tryptophan operon can be most easily detected by

(A) Detecting a normal repressor protein by Western blot
(B) Finding intracellular tryptophan metabolites
(C) Growing it in a tryptophan-depleted medium
(D) Noticing increased uptake of labeled tryptophan from the medium
(E) Observing a change in the molecular weight of the repressor gene by Northern blot

43. Of the following clinical manifestations of *S. pneumoniae*, which is the most important as a cause of morbidity and mortality in an older adult?

(A) Endocarditis
(B) Meningitis
(C) Otitis media
(D) Pneumonia
(E) Septic shock

44. In a serum inhibition test, the serum from a patient with toxic shock syndrome receiving intravenous ceftriaxone was found to inhibit the growth of *Staphylococcus aureus* at a dilution of 1:50. The lowest concentration of ceftriaxone that would inhibit growth is 0.75 U/mL. What must be the minimum level of the patient's serum ceftriaxone?

(A) 0.02 U/mL
(B) 0.75 U/mL
(C) 37.5 U/mL
(D) 87.5 U/mL
(E) 100 U/mL

45. *S. pneumoniae* can be distinguished from other streptococci by its

(A) Ability to grow in 6% NaCl
(B) Pattern of red cell lysis
(C) Resistance to bile
(D) Resistance to penicillin
(E) Susceptibility to optochin

46. In a patient with gram-negative sepsis, which of the following is believed to cause fever?

(A) A direct effect of endotoxin on the hypothalamic temperature regulation center
(B) An increased blood supply to the hypothalamus caused by vasoactive mediators
(C) The generation of pyrogenic complement fragments by macrophage proteases
(D) The release of reactive proteins with pyrogenic properties by the liver
(E) The release of TNF-α , IL-1β, and IL-6 by endotoxin-activated macrophages

47. Protective immunity against *Streptococcus pyogenes* is mediated by antibodies reacting with

(A) Capsular polysaccharide
(B) M protein
(C) Protein G
(D) Pyrogenic exotoxin A
(E) Streptolysin O

48. An alginate-producing, aerobe, oxidase-positive, gram-negative rod was isolated from the sputum of a patient with cystic fibrosis. This organism is likely to be

(A) *Bacteroides fragilis*
(B) *E. coli*
(C) *Klebsiella pneumoniae*
(D) *Pseudomonas aeruginosa*
(E) *Streptococcus faecalis*

49. Which of the following infections is acquired through lice?

(A) Bartonellosis
(B) Ehrlichiosis
(C) Epidemic typhus
(D) Lyme disease
(E) Q fever

50. The production of urease by *H. pylori* is biologically relevant because it

(A) Allows *H. pylori* to use urea as a nutrient
(B) Generates ammonia, which causes tissue damage
(C) Is the basis for a rapid diagnostic test for *H. pylori*
(D) Protects *H. pylori* against the extremely low pH of its environment
(E) Raises the pH of the urine

51. If a vaccine was to be developed to prevent intestinal colonization of *E. coli,* which of the following bacterial structures should be presented to the mucosal immune system?

(A) Capsular polysaccharide
(B) Fimbriae
(C) Lipopolysaccharide
(D) Peptidoglycan
(E) Teichoic acid

52. Based on their mechanisms of action, which one of the following antibiotics would you predict has the lowest toxicity for humans?

(A) Aminoglycosides
(B) β-lactams
(C) Fluoroquinolones
(D) Macrolides
(E) Tetracyclines

53. For decontamination of a heat-sensitive reusable piece of equipment, which ONE of the following procedures would you consider most efficient?

(A) Ethylene oxide gas sterilization
(B) Pasteurization
(C) Soaking in 3% hydrogen peroxide
(D) Soaking in alcohol
(E) Ultraviolet (UV) irradiation

QUESTIONS 54–55

A 5-year-old black boy with a deficiency of the C6 component of the complement system presents with a febrile disease associated with headaches, nuchal rigidity, and decreased alertness. A Gram stain of a cytospin of CSF obtained by lumbar puncture shows gram-negative cocci, predominantly arranged in pairs.

54. Which is the most likely organism involved in this patient's disease?

    (A) *H. influenzae*
    (B) *Neisseria gonorrhoeae*
    (C) *Neisseria meningitidis*
    (D) *Serratia marcescens*
    (E) *S. pneumoniae*

55. The most important virulence factor(s) of this organism is (are) its

    (A) Endotoxin
    (B) Neurotoxin
    (C) Penicillinase-coding plasmids
    (D) Polysaccharide capsule
    (E) Superantigenic exotoxins

56. After ingestion by macrophages, which of the following mechanisms is believed to be responsible for the survival of mycobacteria?

    (A) Inactivation of oxygen active radicals
    (B) Induction of a state of unresponsiveness to activating cytokines
    (C) Inhibition of phagolysosome formation
    (D) Rapid escape from the phagosomes into the cytoplasm
    (E) Resistance of the mycobacterial cell wall against superoxide and nitric oxide

QUESTIONS 57–58

After a cesarean section, a 36-year-old woman becomes febrile, complains of a tender abdomen, and exhibits a foul-smelling vaginal discharge. An emergency magnetic resonance image (MRI) of the abdomen is compatible with a periuterine gas-containing abscess. Blood tests are as follows: complete blood count (CBC) shows anemia with poikilocytosis and moderate reticulocytosis; WBC count is 15,000/ L with 69% neutrophils and 13% bands. Serum haptoglobin is low.

57. The organism most likely responsible for this clinical picture is

    (A) *Bacteroides fragilis*
    (B) *Clostridium difficile*
    (C) *Clostridium perfringens*
    (D) *Fusobacterium nucleatum*
    (E) *Peptostreptococcus asaccharolyticus*

58. The organism most likely involved secretes a major exotoxin that

    (A) Blocks neuromuscular transmission
    (B) Cleaves peptide bonds
    (C) Hydrolyzes phospholipids, such as lecithin
    (D) Inhibits protein synthesis
    (E) Solubilizes collagen

QUESTIONS 59–60

A 4-year-old toddler became ill with bloody diarrhea within 48 hours of eating a hamburger at a fast food shop. Initial culture of his bloody stool revealed a gram-negative, lactose fermenter, indole-positive rod. A filtrate to the stool was put on Vero cells and cytotoxicity occurred within 24 hours.

59. Which of the following complications could develop in the course of this patient's disease?

    (A) Enteric fever
    (B) Hemolytic-uremic syndrome
    (C) Intestinal perforation
    (D) Septic shock
    (E) Toxic shock syndrome

60. The virulence factor responsible for this patient's disease is very similar to a virulence factor characteristic of

    (A) *Corynebacterium diphtheriae*
    (B) *Neisseria meningitidis*
    (C) *Shigella dysenteriae*
    (D) *Shigella flexneri*
    (E) *Vibrio cholerae*

61. A 70-year-old man suffering from renal insufficiency is admitted to the hospital mentally confused, complaining of shortness of breath, and having a productive cough. His temperature is 102°F. A blood count reveals 13,000 WBCs/mm^3, with a differential analysis of 70% neutrophils and 15% lymphocytes. A sputum Gram stain reveals gram-positive cocci arranged in pairs. Which of the following measures could have prevented this disease?

    (A) Better treatment of his kidney insufficiency
    (B) Immunization
    (C) Isolation from individuals with the same disease
    (D) Prophylactic administration of gamma globulin
    (E) Prophylactic administration of slow-release penicillin

QUESTIONS 62–63

A 37-year-old Mexican migrant farm worker is admitted because of muscle spasms. He has pharyngeal spasms when he tries to swallow and general rigidity of all muscles. When stimulated by loud noises he has severe generalized muscle spasms, opisthotonos, and risus sardonicus.

62. Which is the mechanism of action of the virulence factor responsible for this patient's symptoms?

 (A) Hydrolysis of lecithin and sphingomyelin-containing phospholipids
 (B) Increased activity of the autonomic hypothalamic nuclei
 (C) Inhibition of the release of neurologic inhibitory transmitters
 (D) Interference with the release of acetylcholine at the neuromuscular junctions
 (E) Stimulation of the motor neurons

63. The organism responsible for this disease can be described as

 (A) Gram-negative, aerobic rod
 (B) Gram-negative, spore-forming, anaerobic rod
 (C) Gram-positive, anaerobic rod
 (D) Gram-positive, spore-forming, aerobic rod
 (E) Gram-positive, spore-forming, anaerobic rod

64. A patient is seen 4 days after a dental extraction with a draining, suppurative abscess in the soft tissues of the lower jaw. A gram-positive, branching, filamentous anaerobic organism is isolated. This organism most likely belongs to the genus

 (A) *Actinomyces*
 (B) *Mycobacterium*
 (C) *Nocardia*
 (D) *Staphylococcus*
 (E) *Streptomyces*

65. Methicillin resistance in *Staphylococcus aureus* is accounted for by which of the following mechanisms?

 (A) Active excretion of penicillin
 (B) Impermeability of the outer membrane
 (C) Mutations on the penicillin-binding proteins
 (D) Synthesis of a β-lactamase active against **all** β-lactam antibiotics
 (E) Synthesis of a β-lactamase active mostly against methicillin

66. Which of the following bacteria is strictly transmitted from humans to other humans, without participation of animal reservoirs in the chain of transmission?

 (A) *Campylobacter jejuni*
 (B) *E. coli* O157:H7
 (C) *H. influenzae* type B
 (D) *Listeria monocytogenes*
 (E) *Salmonella enteritidis*

67. Disseminated intravascular coagulation associated with bacterial infections is primarily caused by

 (A) Disseminated endothelial damage
 (B) Generalized activation of infected macrophages
 (C) Intravascular activation of the complement system
 (D) Massive release of endotoxin
 (E) Release of proteases from infected cells which activate the clotting system

QUESTIONS 68–69

A 28-year-old woman is admitted to the emergency room with intense pain caused by kidney stones. A freshly collected clean catch urine sample was cloudy, alkaline (pH 8.6), and the sediment contained numerous polymorphonuclear leukocytes and an average of eight bacteria per high-power field. A Gram stain of the urinary sediment characterized the bacteria as gram-negative rods.

68. This patient most likely has an infection with

 (A) *E. coli*
 (B) *Klebsiella pneumoniae*
 (C) *Proteus mirabilis*
 (D) *Pseudomonas aeruginosa*
 (E) *Serratia marcescens*

69. The colonies of the agent involved in this patient's urinary tract infection are characteristically described as

 (A) Hemolytic
 (B) Mucoid
 (C) Pigmented
 (D) Smooth
 (E) Swarming

70. A 2-day-old infant is admitted with fever, hypotension, and respiratory difficulties. Blood cultures revealed a catalase-negative, β-hemolytic, bacitracin-resistant, gram-positive coccus. This pathogen is most likely

 (A) *E. coli*
 (B) Group B *Streptococcus*
 (C) *Listeria monocytogenes*
 (D) *Moraxella catarrhalis*
 (E) *Streptococcus pyogenes*

71. Development of poststreptococcal glomerulonephritis is believed to be caused by

(A) Bacteremia and secondary infection of the renal parenchyma

(B) Glomerular endothelial damage caused by endotoxin

(C) Red cell hemolysis and secondary renal damage

(D) Release of a nephritogenic toxin from infected tissues

(E) Synthesis of cross-reactive antibodies that react with glomerular antigens

72. The ability of group A streptococci to cause pyogenic infections is DIRECTLY related to the production of

(A) Erythrogenic toxin

(B) Hyaluronidase

(C) M protein

(D) Streptokinase

(E) Streptolysin O

73. Which ONE of the following virulence factors is common to *Neisseria, S. pneumoniae,* and *H. influenzae?*

(A) β-lactamases

(B) IgA protease

(C) Lipopolysaccharide

(D) Protein A

(E) Protein G

74. A strain of *E. coli* which is positive for the *lac* operon (*lac*⁺) and penicillin resistant (pen^R) can transfer these traits to *lac*-negative (*lac*−), penicillin-susceptible (pen^S) strains. All the recipient bacteria become pen^R but only about half become simultaneously *lac*⁺, pen^R. The recipient bacteria can transfer their newly acquired traits to other *lac*− pen^S strains. The isolated transfer of the *lac*⁺ trait is not observed in this experiment. The transfer process is not affected by DNAse added to the medium but is inhibited if the strains are incubated in 2 communicating chambers separated by a 0.4 m filter which excludes bacteria (but not viruses). These observations suggest that

(A) A plasmid coding for pen^R mobilized a second plasmid coding for *lac*⁺

(B) The pen^R and *lac*⁺ traits are transmitted independently by transformation

(C) The pen^R and *lac*⁺ traits were transferred by Hfr recombination

(D) The simultaneous transmission of the genes coding for pen^R and *lac*⁺ requires two phage populations, each one carrying one gene

75. Gram-positive bacteria uniquely contain

(A) Lipopolysaccharide

(B) Peptidoglycan

(C) Polysaccharide capsule

(D) Porins

(E) Teichoic acid

76. What is the nature of the immunizing agent(s) contained in the acellular pertussis vaccine?

(A) Attenuated bacteria

(B) Bacterial DNA

(C) Inactive toxin + adhesion factor(s)

(D) Polysaccharide

(E) Killed bacteria

(F) Polysaccharide-toxoid conjugate

(G) Synthetic peptides

(H) Toxoid

77. A 4-year-old boy is admitted to the hospital with shortness of breath, a productive cough, and a temperature of 104°F which had been preceded by a sudden and hard rigor. A blood count revealed 20,000 WBC/mL, with a differential analysis of 75% neutrophils and 20% lymphocytes. A Gram stain of the sputum showed extracellular gram-negative coccobacilli that grew well in chocolate agar but not in blood agar. This infection could have been prevented by immunization with

(A) Attenuated bacteria

(B) Killed bacteria

(C) Polysaccharide

(D) Polysaccharide-toxo...

(E) Recombinant bacteri...

(F) Recombinant protein

(G) Synthetic peptide

(H) Toxoid

78. An 18-year-old boy present... ...arged, hot, red, and painful adenopathy in th... left axilla associated with a temperature of 102°F. A serological test for antibodies to *Bartonella henselae* is positive. This infection was likely transmitted by

(A) Cat scratch

(B) Dog bite

(C) Droplet inhalation

(D) Ingestion of contaminated food

(E) Mosquito bite

(F) Rodent urine

(G) Sexual intercourse

(H) Tick bite

79. A 70-year-old veteran with chronic bronchitis is hospitalized after being seen at the emergency room with productive cough, fever (104°F), and diarrhea. A chest radiograph was compatible with bilateral bronchopneumonia. A Gram stain and culture of the sputum and a stool culture failed to yield any pathogenic bacteria but cultures in charcoal-yeast agar supplemented with cysteine were positive. The organism responsible for this infection is

(A) *Bacteroides fragilis*
(B) *Bartonella (Rochalimaea) henselae*
(C) *Chlamydia pneumoniae*
(D) *Chlamydia psittaci*
(E) *Francisella tularensis*
(F) *H. influenzae*
(G) *Legionella pneumophila*
(H) *Mycobacterium tuberculosis*
(I) *Mycoplasma pneumoniae*
(J) *S. pneumoniae*

Directions: (Items 80–85) Each of the numbered items or incomplete statements in this section is negatively phrased, as indicated by a capitalized word such as NOT, LEAST, or EXCEPT. Select the ONE lettered answer or completion that is BEST in each case.

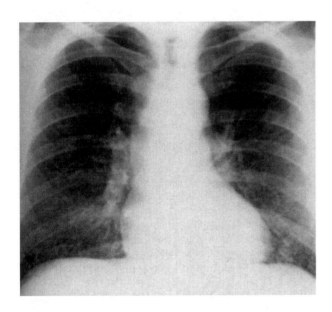

80. A 15-year-old boy complains of fever, headaches, and persistent unproductive cough for the last 4 days. Lung auscultation reveals rhonchi and rales in both bases. The chest radiograph is shown in the figure. A cold agglutinin test is positive. Blood culture and additional serological studies are pending. Which of the following types of antibiotics will be the LEAST indicated to start treatment in this patient?

(A) An inhibitor of peptidoglycan cross-linking
(B) An inhibitor of dihydrofolate reductase
(C) A DNA synthesis inhibitor
(D) A protein synthesis inhibitor
(E) A transcription inhibitor

81. All of the following are important tests to carry out in a case of intra-abdominal abscess EXCEPT

(A) Gram stain
(B) Aerobic cultures
(C) Anaerobic cultures
(D) Tests for enterotoxins
(E) Antibiotic susceptibility tests

82. In a patient with food poisoning caused by *Clostridium botulinum*, which symptom is LEAST often observed?

(A) Double vision
(B) Dysphagia
(C) Respiratory paralysis
(D) Severe diarrhea
(E) Urinary retention

83. To demonstrate linkage between 2 chromosomal genes in a given bacterium, which of the following genetic processes is LEAST useful?

(A) Generalized transduction
(B) Hfr conjugation
(C) Specialized transduction
(D) Transformation

84. All of the following characteristics of a gram-negative organism may be plasmid-coded, EXCEPT

(A) Antibiotic resistance
(B) Conjugating ability
(C) Expression of adhesion factors
(D) Lipopolysaccharide toxicity
(E) Synthesis of enterotoxins

85. A healthy 12-month-old boy has a brother with adenosine deaminase deficiency. Which of the following vaccines should you NOT administer to the infant?

(A) Diphtheria-tetanus-pertussis (DTP)
(B) *H. influenzae* (HiB)
(C) Hepatitis B (Hep B)
(D) Oral polio vaccine
(E) Measles-mumps-rubella (MMR)

TEST 2: Bacteriology

1. A	18. D	35. E	52. B	69. E
2. A	19. C	36. B	53. A	70. B
3. C	20. D	37. E	54. C	71. E
4. D	21. A	38. B	55. A	72. C
5. B	22. D	39. A	56. C	73. B
6. B	23. A	40. D	57. C	74. A
7. A	24. C	41. C	58. C	75. E
8. D	25. C	42. C	59. B	76. C
9. E	26. B	43. D	60. C	77. D
10. E	27. B	44. C	61. B	78. A
11. E	28. D	45. E	62. C	79. G
12. D	29. B	46. E	63. E	80. A
13. B	30. C	47. B	64. A	81. D
14. C	31. C	48. D	65. C	82. D
15. E	32. E	49. C	66. C	83. C
16. B	33. B	50. D	67. A	84. D
17. D	34. A	51. B	68. C	85. D

ANSWERS AND EXPLANATIONS

Note: Page numbers designated as "IMI 4th Ed" refer to *Introduction to Medical Immunology,* 4th ed., New York/Basel, Marcel Dekker, 1998. Page numbers designated as "NMS M&ID 3rd Ed" refer to *NMS Microbiology and Infectious Diseases,* 3rd ed. Baltimore, Williams & Wilkins, 1997. Page numbers indicated as "PAInfDis4th Ed" refer to Reese RE, Betts RF, eds., *Practical Approach to Infectious Diseases,* 4th ed., Boston, Little, Brown & Co., 1996.

1. The answer is A. This question is best addressed by elimination. Transformation, mediated by soluble DNA transfer from cell to cell, would be affected by DNAse in the medium. Transduction (i.e., transfer of genetic material by bacteriophages) is ruled out by the fact that the process was inhibited by filters that did not exclude viruses. Conjugation involving an Hfr strain does not usually result in acquisition of the fertility factor, and therefore, transmission from bacteria to bacteria of the *lac+* trait would be highly unlikely. The best scenario is conjugation involving an F⁺ plasmid carrying the resistance gene. All the details of the experiment fit in this hypothesis. (NMS M&ID, 3rd Ed. p. 28–34)

2. The answer is A. Duffy red cell antigen is the receptor for *Plasmodium vivax,* one of the sporozoans that causes malaria. ICAM-1 is the receptor for rhinoviruses in the nasal mucosa. Outer membrane proteins interact, among others, with the fertility factor of F⁺ bacteria. Sialated Lewis[b] antigen has been identified as the receptor for *H. pylori.*(NMS M&ID, 3rd Ed. p. 152).

3. The answer is C. Only lysogenized *Corynebacterium diphtheriae* strains produce diphtheria toxin, which is coded by a gene (*tox*) carried by the integrated prophage. The gene expression is controlled by a bacterial repressor, which is regulated by the availability of iron in the medium. When iron concentrations become too low, the gene is expressed. The cleavage of the toxin happens after secretion, and the change from lysogenic to lytic infection is not necessary for *tox* gene expression. (NMS M&ID, 3rd Ed. p. 113)

4. The answer is D. The clinical picture is strongly suggestive of pseudomembranous colitis, which is caused by the overgrowth of *Clostridium difficile* (a gram-positive rod that secretes two potent cytotoxins, A and B) in patients receiving broad-spectrum antibiotics—particularly clindamycin, ampicillin, and cephalosporins. (NMS M&ID, 3rd Ed. p. 119–20)

5. The answer is B. Because plasmids contain accessory genetic information, they are not present in all members of a bacterial species; they actually account for differences in virulence between isolates from the same species. Plasmid-coded virulence factors include enzymes, toxins, and adhesion factors, and can be expressed constitutively or only in special conditions, such as under metabolic stress. (NMS M&ID, 3rd Ed. p. 34–5, 65–70)

6. The answer is B. The case description should raise the suspicion of cat-scratch disease as the most likely diagnosis, because of the typical clinical presentation and the child has contact with domestic cats. Cat scratch disease is caused by *Bartonella henselae.* Though related, *Bartonella bacilliformis* causes bartonellosis and is transmitted by insect bites. The only other organism that can be transmitted by cats is *Pasteurella multocida,* but usually after a bite. *Francisella tularensis* can be transmitted by scratch, but from rabbits, not cats. *Yersinia pestis* is transmitted by the rat flea. (NMS M&ID, 3rd Ed. p. 166, 201–2)

7. The answer is A. The 16S ribosomal RNA gene codes for a structural component that is essential for protein synthesis. There are regions on the gene that are subject to genetic drift; that is, they can vary without affecting protein synthesis because they do not affect the spatial folding of the 16S ribosome, which is what determines its ability to participate in protein synthesis. Hence, these sequences reflect evolutionary distance and species identity and because the gene is small (~1600 base pairs) they are much easier to determine than the complete genome sequences. It must also be noted that ribosomal RNA genes are found in every living creature, including prokaryotes, archeobacteria, and eukaryotes. All other choices lack specificity, compared with nucleic acid sequences.

8. The answer is D. In a newborn with meningitis, the recovery of a gram-positive pleomorphic rod suggests that *Listeria monocytogenes* is the responsible organism (other rods that could be involved—Enterobacteriaceae and *H. influenzae*—are gram-negative). The remaining characteristics, catalase positivity and microaerophilic growth, are characteristic of this organism. β-lactam antibiotics, which interfere with peptidoglycan cross-linking, are the drugs of choice for this organism, which has never been reported to acquire penicillin resistance. (NMS M&ID, 3rd Ed. p. 116–7)

9. The answer is E. *H. influenzae* was the most common bacterial cause of meningitis in young children, but the incidence of meningitis caused by this organism has sharply declined after the introduction of the conjugate vaccines. The cases seen at the present time are caused by *N. meningitidis* or *S. pneumoniae*. Group B *Streptococcus* and *E. coli* are commonly involved in neonatal bacteremia and meningitis, but are not a problem in children past the first month of life. Group A *Streptococcus* is not usually recovered from patients with meningitis at any age. (NMS M&ID, 3rd Ed. p. 85, 135–6, 431–3)

10. The answer is E. *Salmonella enteritidis* species are not usually involved in systemic infections, but the exception is patients with sickle cell anemia. As a consequence of multiple and repeated splenic infarcts during sickling crises, the splenic tissue is replaced by nonfunctional fibrotic tissue. The loss of splenic function is associated with persistence of bacteria in circulation, enhancing the bacteria's opportunity to infect a variety of organs and tissues. For reasons that are not entirely clear, *S. enteritidis* is the most frequent agent involved as the cause of osteomyelitis in these patients. All other listed infections are caused by pathogenic bacteria in immunocompetent individuals. (IMI 4th Ed., p. 602–3; NMS M&ID, 3rd Ed., p. 149; PAInfDis 4th Ed., p. 608)

11. The answer is E. Among the diseases transmitted by ticks, Rocky Mountain spotted fever is more prevalent in the Southeast United States. Diagnosis may be difficult in the early stages of the disease, but in this case it should be suspected because of the history of a tick bite in the woods. It is important to start therapy as early as possible, because the disease can be fatal, and delay in treatment is associated with increased fatality rates. The drugs of choice are the tetracyclines and chloramphenicol, the former preferred based on its lower toxicity. It must also be noted that tetracyclines are effective against most bacterial infections transmitted by ticks, including the rickettsioses and Lyme disease. (NMS M&ID, 3rd Ed. p. 181–3, 198–200)

12. The answer is D. Rickettsiae are obligatory intracellular parasites because they require growth factors provided by the infected cells. Although they are structurally similar to gram-negative organisms (their cell wall contains lipopolysaccharides), they stain poorly, and cannot be visualized by a Gram stain. Rocky Mountain spotted fever is not an opportunistic infection; it usually affects previously healthy individuals. (NMS M&ID, 3rd Ed. p. 181–3, 198)

13. The answer is B. The case history corresponds to a patient with typhoid fever. However, it is difficult to make the diagnosis based exclusively on clinical information. But the constellation of symptoms—fever and maculopapular rash—suggest a systemic infection, and blood cultures appear to be the best starting point in an attempt to diagnose this patient's disease. Biopsy of skin lesions could be considered, but only in addition to blood cultures. The same rationale would apply to serological tests for brucellosis. Viral diseases such as measles or rubella are seen in children; it would be very rare to have two adults suffering from such diseases at the same time, in the same community. (NMS M&ID, 3rd Ed. p. 149–50)

14. The answer is C. The scenario is clearly that of a food poisoning case, probably involving ingestion of a preformed toxin a few hours before the symptoms started. The travel history is not relevant, because there is no known infectious agent that would cause this type of food poisoning 14 days after ingestion. The possibility of having brought contaminated food from the trip cannot be totally ruled out, but it is rather unlikely, considering that it is illegal for travelers to bring food into the country. (NMS M&ID, 3rd Ed. p. 455–62)

15. The answer is E. An acute gastroenteritis with profuse diarrhea and vomiting is typically caused by ingestion of a preformed toxin. *Staphylococcus aureus* should be a very likely candidate. This bacterium is, by far, the most frequent cause of this type of food poisoning, and vomiting is a prominent feature because one of the staphylococcal enterotoxins—enterotoxin A—stimulates the vomit center through neural receptors in the upper gastrointestinal tract, hence not in the villi or the mucosa of the small intestine. (NMS M&ID, 3rd Ed. p. 102–4; 460). In the author's experience, allergic reactions to food may be associated with anaphylactic shock or hives, perhaps in some cases with diarrhea, but their onset is faster and vomiting is not one of the symptoms.

16. The answer is B. Several infectious agents can cause relapsing or recurrent fevers. *Chlamydia psittaci, Bartonella henselae,* and *Pasteurella multocida* are not associated with sheep. *Brucella abortus* and *Coxiella burnetii* are zoonotic bacteria and both can be acquired from sheep. *Brucella* is usually acquired by ingesting infected milk or cheese and the resulting disease is characterized by recurrent fever; pneumonia is not a prominent feature. *Coxiella,* in contrast, is acquired by inhalation and pulmonary symptomatology is almost always present. Treatment of both infections with most antibiotics is ineffective, perhaps because these two organisms proliferate intracellularly (*Coxiella* is an obligatory intracellular organism, *Brucella* is a facultative intracellular organism). The drugs of choice for both organisms are the tetracyclines, none of which were used to treat the patient. (NMS M&ID, 3rd Ed. p. 162–4, 198–201)

17. The answer is D. When lactose is not needed because of the easy availability of glucose, the *lac* operon remains silent. Lactose is taken up in concentrations sufficient to inactivate the repressor, but the expression of the *lac* gene does not take place because a catabolite activator protein (CAP), essential for transcription of the operon, cannot bind to the operator region. This is a consequence of the CAP protein only being able to bind to the promoter region in the presence of cAMP, and the levels of cAMP being very low when glucose is used. The expression of the catabolite repressor gene is constitutive, not influenced by variations in sugar levels. (NMS M&ID, 3rd Ed. p. 36–8)

18. The answer is D. The patient has a urinary tract infection (UTI). Because the patient has fever and flank pain, and granular casts have been detected in her urine, the infection has reached the kidney, and therefore a diagnosis of pyelonephritis should be considered. *E. coli* is the most common cause of community-acquired UTIs, and it fits the data given: gram-negative rod, lactose fermenter, indole-positive. The strains that cause pyelonephritis have a special "P" fimbriae which enable the organisms to attach to the epithelial lining of the upper urinary tract. Unique O antigens appear to be expressed by strains that infect the lower urinary tract (bladder and urethra).(NMS M&ID, 3rd Ed. p. 144)

19. The answer is C. Most infectious agents that cause recurrent fevers do so by undergoing sequential antigenic mutations. The immune system responds to each mutant and the patient appears to recover, but relapses with the emergence of a new antigenic mutant, which is not affected by the preformed antibodies to previous mutants. This is known as "antigenic variation" and has been well characterized for *Borrelia recurrentis,* trypanosomes, *Plasmodium falciparum,* HIV, and several other infectious agents. Intracellular sequestration by itself could not explain the recurrence of fever. (NMS M&ID, 3rd Ed. p. 79–80, 180, 266)

20. The answer is D. Impetigo is caused by two grampositive cocci, *Staphylococcus aureus* and *Streptococcus pyogenes*. Both organisms have in common a thick peptidoglycan layer in their cell wall, typical of grampositive organisms. Both organisms are easy to grow in conventional media and *S. pyogenes* can grow anaerobically. These organisms have a variety of virulence factors, but polysaccharide capsules are not among them. (NMS M&ID, 3rd Ed. p. 7, 101–7)

21. The answer is A. *Staphylococcus aureus* is frequently resistant to β-lactams due to the synthesis of plasmid-coded β-lactamases. None of the other resistance mechanisms applies to this organism.(NMS M&ID, 3rd Ed. p. 55)

22. The answer is D. Skin infections by *Streptococcus pyogenes* can be followed by poststreptococcal glomerulonephritis, probably resulting from the synthesis of cross-reactive antibodies reacting with antigens of the kidney basement membrane. Another nonsuppurative complication of streptococcal infection is rheumatic fever, of which carditis and arthritis may be part, but it is usually seen after throat infections, and its frequency has declined significantly. Erysipelas and toxic shock are manifestations of an ongoing infection. (NMS M&ID, 3rd Ed. p. 109)

23. The answer is A. Macrolide antibiotics (e.g., erythromycin) inhibit protein synthesis by causing premature chain termination. Thus, leucine incorporation would be inhibited. Lack of thymine incorporation would indicate that the antibiotic interfered with DNA synthesis, in the same way that lack of uracil incorporation would imply interference with RNA synthesis. Lack of incorporation of ribose would indicate interference with glycosylation, a mechanism of action that has not been described for any antimicrobial agent. (NMS M&ID, 3rd Ed. p. 51)

24. The answer is C. Ciprofloxacin is a fluoroquinolone and this group of antibacterial agents interferes with the function of DNA gyrase. Therefore, DNA gyrase mutations can potentially result in a functional enzyme with decreased affinity for fluoroquinolones, and, as a consequence, the organism becomes resistant to this group of antimicrobials. All other listed targets are affected by antibiotics, but not by fluoroquinolones. (NMS M&ID, 3rd Ed. p. 48, 54–7)

25. The answer is C. Most bacterial polysaccharide capsules have antiphagocytic properties; i.e., they confer a charge to the organism that prevents its effective ingestion. Some capsules also have anticomplementary activity, meaning that they block complement activation, preventing the accumulation of active fragments. Polysaccharides are not strongly immunogenic, but in most cases elicit antibody responses that can play a significant role in eventually eliminating the organism and protecting against subsequent infections. The structure of bacterial polysaccharides has no known homology with that of mammalian cell membrane antigens. (NMS M&ID, 3rd Ed. p. 79)

26. The answer is B. The poor immunogenicity of bacterial polysaccharides is more manifest in young children than in adults. Therefore, children often fail to develop protective antibodies. This problem can be solved by administering conjugate vaccines, prepared by coupling bacterial polysaccharides to protein carriers, such as bacterial toxoids or membrane proteins. Such conjugate vaccines function much as hapten-carrier conjugates and elicit strong immune responses to polysaccharides, even in young children. Such conjugate vaccines for *S. pneumoniae* are currently being tested. None of the other alternatives are as likely to be useful for efficient vaccination against *S. pneumoniae*. Efficient mucosal stimulation would require the development of attenuated strains; more potent adjuvants would induce strong inflammatory reactions at the site of injections. Using whole killed bacteria or increasing the number of strains in the vaccine would not solve the problem of poor immunogenicity. (NMS M&ID, 3rd Ed. p. 84–5; IMI 4th Ed., p. 55–8, 230)

27. The answer is B. The experimental conditions described were such that the two populations of *E. coli* would be able to proliferate and exchange genetic information by high-frequency recombination (transformation was prevented by adding DNAse to the medium). The fact that some tetracycline (tet)-resistant organisms required tryptophan (trp) but not histidine (his) for growth proves that there was genetic exchange between the two strains, with transfer of the tet-resistance gene from the resistant strain to the susceptible strain. The fact that all auxotrophic tet-resistant strains required trp for growth, but only 40% required both trp and his, proves that the his gene must be closer to the tet-resistance gene than the trp gene. (NMS M&ID, 3rd Ed. p. 84–85; IMI 4th Ed., p. 55–8, 230)

28. The answer is D. The nitroimidazoles become active after reduction of their 5-nitro group; the reduced form alkylates DNA and causes strand breaks, thus interfering with DNA replication. The reduction of nitroimidazoles only takes place in anaerobic bacteria, which use low redox potential compounds as electron acceptors; these are the compounds that eventually reduce the nitroimidazoles. (NMS M&ID, 3rd Ed. p. 48)

29. The answer is B. Perú is the epicenter of an ongoing cholera epidemic, and that fact, associated with profuse watery diarrhea of acute onset, are sufficient to establish a presumptive diagnosis of cholera. *Vibrio cholerae* causes diarrhea by releasing a toxin that ribosylates a Gs protein associated with adenylate cyclase, which becomes activated and generates high levels of intracellular cAMP. This, in turn, leads to increased electrolyte flux into the intestinal lumen, and the hypertonicity of the intestinal contents causes water transport, and from that results the watery diarrhea. All other choices correspond to mechanisms of diarrhea caused by other organisms. (NMS M&ID, 3rd Ed. p. 144–54)

30. The answer is C. Component vaccines, such as those listed in the five answers, are usually prepared using either inactivated toxins (toxoids, recombinant toxins), capsular polysaccharides, or adhesion factors. The first prevent the manifestations of the disease, the second override the antiphagocytic effects of bacterial capsules, and the third prevent colonization. In the case of *H. pylori* the best strategy would probably be to induce immunity against adhesion factors (such as the adhesin that binds to the *H. pylori* receptor, sialated Lewis[b] blood group antigen), trying to prevent the bacteria from infecting the host. The in vivo effects of vacuolating cytotoxin A are ill-defined and believed to be strictly local, so a vaccine against this component does not appear as appealing. Note that *H. pylori* does not have an IgA protease. (NMS M&ID, 3rd Ed. p. 84–5, 156–7)

31. The answer is C. The American Academy of Pediatrics and other professional organizations have recommended that the hepatitis B vaccine be administered to all newborns immediately after birth in an effort to cut down perinatal transmission of the virus. There is no approved HIV vaccine, and all other vaccines listed are given in the usual schedule, starting at 2 months of age. (NMS M&ID, 3rd Ed. p. 86)

32. The answer is E. The characteristics of the organisms isolated from the patient's urine allow its identification as *Pseudomonas aeruginosa.* This organism is often acquired as a consequence of bladder catheterization. *Klebsiella* colonies are also mucoid, but this organism is oxidase-negative and does not release a green pigment. The remaining organisms do not share any of the described properties of *Pseudomonas.* (NMS M&ID, 3rd Ed. p. 160–2)

33. The answer is B. The listed characteristics of the organism allow its identification as *Staphylococcus aureus,* which often produces β-lactamases. *S. aureus* is not a facultative intracellular organism; it does not have endotoxin on its cell wall, and none of its exotoxins can be described as a neurotoxin. Glomerulonephritis is associated with streptococcal infections. (NMS M&ID, 3rd Ed. p. 101–2)

34. The answer is A. The organism most likely to be acquired through a skin abrasion on a freshwater tank is *Mycobacterium marinum,* an acid-fast rod that grows better at 30°C. *Pseudomonas* can also survive as a free-living organism in water, but it will cause a purulent lesion, rather than a granulomatous infection, as suggested by the nodular characteristics of this patient's lesion. (NMS M&ID, 3rd Ed. p. 171–2)

35. The answer is E. *Mycobacterium marinum* is susceptible to tetracyclines, trimethoprim-sulfonamide, and to the usual antituberculous drugs (such as rifampin, isoniazid, and clarithromycin), but when the lesion is limited to the skin, excision is effective and avoids the use of antibiotics for a prolonged time. (NMS M&ID, 3rd Ed. p. 172)

36. The answer is B. The clinical case is suggestive of legionnaires' disease—a 73-year-old smoker who develops what appears to be a bacterial pneumonia associated with diarrhea, with negative Gram and acid-fast stains. *Legionella pneumophila* does not stain with the conventional Gram stain and is difficult to isolate, so often treatment has to be started empirically, and it is important to know that the drugs of choice are the macrolides, such as erythromycin. Doxycycline is a broad-spectrum tetracycline; isoniazid is used to treat tuberculosis; metronidazole is used to treat parasitic or anaerobic bacterial infections; penicillin G is mostly active against gram-positive staphylococci and streptococci. (NMS M&ID, 3rd Ed. p. 185–7)

37. The answer is E. Of the listed media, charcoal-yeast extract with cysteine is the best for growing *Legionella,* but other possibilities could not be totally eliminated, so cultures in a variety of media should be seeded. Blood agar is a good general medium on which many organisms (including *S. pneumoniae*) will grow; chocolate agar is the medium for *H. influenzae,* and the Lowenstein-Jensen culture medium is adequate for *Mycobacterium tuberculosis.* Thayer-Martin agar, in contrast, is the medium of choice for growing *N. gonorrhoeae* from samples contaminated with normal flora, and the involvement of this organism in a pulmonary infection is extremely unlikely. (NMS M&ID, 3rd Ed. p. 95, 185–7)

38. The answer is B. An enzyme immunoassay for *Legionella* antigens in the urine has been recently described with high sensitivity and specificity and is becoming the technique of choice for confirming the diagnosis of legionnaires' disease. The results with this technique are not faster than those obtained with any of the other techniques that can be used, i.e., cultures of biopsy tissue in charcoal-yeast extract with cysteine or direct immunofluorescence using anti-*Legionella* antibodies, but they are more frequently positive and false-positives appear not to occur. Treatment still needs to be initiated before the diagnosis is confirmed. Note that any assay based on the detection of specific antibodies may require testing of two samples (acute and convalescent), an additional complicating factor. Although diarrhea is a common feature, isolation from fecal material has not been reported (the medium should be charcoal-yeast ex-

tract with cysteine, not MacConkey), and methenamine-silver stain will reveal *Pneumocystis carinii* and other fungi, but is not adequate for *Legionella.* (NMS M&ID, 3rd Ed. p. 95, 185–7)

39. The answer is A. The characteristics of the isolated organism are typical of *Neisseria meningitidis.* This gram-negative coccus releases a potent endotoxin that causes extremely severe forms of septic shock associated with a high mortality rate. Dissemination through bacteremia and possible neurologic sequelae of meningococcal meningitis are also cause of concern, but these are not as immediate concerns as the risk of developing septic shock. Most common antimicrobials are effective (e.g., penicillins, cephalosporins) and so this is not a concern. (NMS M&ID, 3rd Ed. p. 125–8, 414)

40. The answer is D. *Neisseria meningitidis* continues to be extremely susceptible to penicillin G, which blocks the cross-linking of bacterial peptidoglycan. If therapy has to be initiated before the organism is identified, a third-generation cephalosporin (which has the same mechanism of action as penicillin G) is more likely to be used, because it will still be active against *N. meningitidis* but has a better chance of being effective against *S. pneumoniae* and *H. influenzae.* (NMS M&ID, 3rd Ed. p. 125–8, 433)

41. The answer is C. The two *E. coli* strains were equally sensitive to neomycin; therefore, the emergence of neomycin resistance cannot have been a consequence of the transfer of genetic information between the two strains, but rather from a spontaneous mutation. Antibiotics do not induce mutations; their role is to select those mutants that are resistant. (NMS M&ID, 3rd Ed. p. 22, 53–4)

42. The answer is C. An auxotrophic strain of *E. coli* with an inactive tryptophan operon cannot synthesize tryptophan and, therefore, it can only grow when tryptophan is added to the medium. A reverse mutation will result in a population of prototrophic bacteria, identical to the wild type strains of the same organism. Those can be easily detected by their ability to grow in the absence of tryptophan. The other alternatives could probably be used for the purpose of detecting an active tryptophan operon, but they are all more complicated procedures than just growing the organism in the absence of tryptophan. (NMS M&ID, 3rd Ed. p. 22–3)

43. The answer is D. *S. pneumoniae* is also the most frequent cause of meningitis in adults, but the frequency of meningitis is considerably lower than the frequency of pneumonia in individuals of that age group. Endocarditis and otitis media in adults are seldom (if ever) caused by *S. pneumoniae* and septic shock is not associated with *S. pneumoniae* infections.(NMS M&ID, 3rd Ed. p. 110–2)

44. The answer is C. If the minimal inhibitory concentration is 0.75 U/mL and the serum can be diluted 1:50 and still retain its bactericidal activity, that means that the serum contains at least a concentration of 50 × 0.75 U/mL, or 37.5 U/mL. (NMS M&ID, 3rd Ed. p. 58–9)

45. The answer is E. Several simple tests can be used to distinguish *S. pneumoniae* from other streptococci, such as bile solubility (*S. pneumoniae* is solubilized by bile) and susceptibility to optochin. The other listed characteristics are not useful for this purpose, including penicillin resistance, because only 20% to 40% of *S. pneumoniae* isolates are resistant to penicillin. (NMS M&ID, 3rd Ed. p. 110–2)

46. The answer is E. In gram-negative sepsis there is massive activation of macrophages by bacterial endotoxin. The activated macrophages release a variety of cytokines, and three of them—TNFα , IL-1β, and IL-6—have pyrogenic properties, i.e., cause elevation of body temperature. This effect is due to the stimulation of a group of nuclei in the anterior hypothalamus that regulate body temperature. Microbial pyrogens do not seem to have direct effects on the temperature regulation center, and, as a rule, reactive proteins (other than cytokines) are not pyrogenic. (NMS M&ID, 3rd Ed. p. 69–70; IMI 4th Ed., p. 195–7)

47. The answer is B. Protective antibodies against *Streptococcus pyogenes* react with the M protein, which has antiphagocytic and anticomplement activities, and together with the closely related protein F promotes adhesion to the epithelial cells of the oropharynx. Protein G binds to the Fc region of IgM and may also play an antiphagocytic role, but protective antibodies do not recognize it. Pyrogenic exotoxin A is only expressed by lysogenized strains. Streptolysin O is strongly immunogenic, but the antibodies against it are more useful as a diagnostic indicator than as conferring protection. The capsular polysaccharide is the major virulence factor of *S. pneumoniae,* against which protective antibodies are directed. (NMS M&ID, 3rd Ed. p. 66, 105–12)

48. The answer is D. The characteristics of the isolated organism allow its identification as *Pseudomonas aeruginosa,* a very common cause of bronchopulmonary infection in patients with cystic fibrosis. Although *Klebsiella pneumoniae* may cause pneumonia, it is neither oxidase-positive nor particularly associated with cystic fibrosis. The remaining bacteria are not usually seen in the described clinical context; none is either an alginate-producer or oxidase-positive; one is a gram-positive coccus (*Streptococcus*); and one is anaerobic (*Bacteroides*). (NMS M&ID, 3rd Ed. p. 160–2)

49. The answer is C. Bartonellosis is transmitted by *Phlebotomus* flies, ehrlichiosis and Lyme disease are transmitted by ticks, and Q fever is usually acquired by inhalation of aerosolized spore-like forms. (NMS M&ID, 3rd Ed. p. 198–202)

50. The answer is D. The breakdown of urea in the gastric environment is believed to help *H. pylori* to survive in the stomach, because ammonia, generated as a consequence of the breakdown of urea, is a strong base and will neutralize hydrochloric acid. This property is used in several diagnostic tests for *H. pylori* infection, but that use has nothing to do with the biological relevance of this enzyme. The tissue damage associated with *H. pylori* infection is believed to be caused by a vacuolating cytotoxin released by the strains associated with gastric ulcers. *H. pylori* does not infect the urinary tract and the effects of *H. pylori* infection on the pH of the urine are negligible. (NMS M&ID, 3rd Ed. p. 156–7)

51. The answer is B. Specialized fimbriae (also known as colonization factors) mediate the adhesion of *E. coli* to mucosal epithelial cells, which is essential for colonization. The lipopolysaccharide oligosaccharide is believed to play a similar role in the case of strains that infect the urinary bladder. The remaining are structural components that have no role in adhesion or colonization. (NMS M&ID, 3rd Ed. p. 142–4)

52. The answer is B. The target of β-lactams is the bacterial peptidoglycan, a structure that is absent in eukaryotic cells, therefore limiting the possibility that this group of antibiotics may interfere with any essential function of the human cells. In contrast, all of the other antibiotics listed have targets that are not unique to prokaryotic cells: ribosomal units (aminoglycosides, macrolides, tetracyclines) or DNA gyrase (fluoroquinolones). (NMS M&ID, 3rd Ed. p. 43–51)

53. The answer is A. Ethylene oxide gas sterilization is an efficient sterilization technique for heat-sensitive objects. Pasteurization is only effective with fluids, and the remaining techniques listed are rather inefficient. (NMS M&ID, 3rd Ed. p. 61–3)

54. The answer is C. Patients with deficiencies of the terminal components of the complement system (C5–C9) have increased incidence of infections caused by bacteria of the *Neisseria* species. The characteristics of the organism isolated from the CSF of this child, which presents with a clinical picture of meningitis, is compatible with *N. meningitidis* (gram-negative diplo-cocci). *Neisseria gonorrhoeae* would be the best second choice. *H. influenzae* and *Serratia marcescens* are gram-negative rods, and *S. pneumoniae* is a diplococcus, but is a gram-positive coccus. (NMS M&ID, 3rd Ed. p. 126, 431–2)

55. The answer is A. Of all the virulence factors identi-fied for *Neisseria meningitidis*—adhesion factors, poly-saccharide capsule, IgA protease, and endotoxin, the last (endotoxin) appears to be the most important from the pathogenic point of view, because it is responsible for the development of a particularly severe form of septic shock (associated with infections by this organ-ism). *Neisseria* species do not ever produce potent exotoxins and *N. meningitidis* has never been demon-strated to acquire penicillinase-coding plasmids. (NMS M&ID, 3rd Ed. p. 126–7)

56. The answer is C. The sulfatide glycolipids of the mycobacterial cell wall inhibit phagolysosome forma-tion and inhibit intraphagosomal acidification, thus cre-ating conditions favorable for the intracellular survival of phagocytized mycobacteria. Rapid escape from phagosomes and resistance to toxic radicals are mecha-nisms of survival used by other facultative intracellular organisms. (NMS M&ID, 3rd Ed. p. 169)

57. The answer is C. The clinical vignette is suggestive of a postoperative anaerobic infection (foul smell, gas-containing abscess), which is associated with anemia, which appears to be of hemolytic origin (poikilocytosis, reticulocytosis, low haptoglobin). The α-toxin of *Clostridium perfringens* is a lecithinase that can disrupt cell membranes and cause hemolysis. The other listed bacteria are all anaerobic, but none of them could cause hemolysis. (NMS M&ID, 3rd Ed. p. 118–9, 467)

58. The answer is C. See answer for question 62. (NMS M&ID, 3rd Ed. p. 118)

59. The answer is B. The clinical picture is suggestive of food poisoning by a bacterium able to invade or dam-age the intestinal mucosa (leading to bloody diarrhea). The listed characteristics are typical of *E. coli* and be-cause the bacteria releases an exotoxin able to kill Vero cells (Verotoxin), it allows the preliminary identification of the isolate as *E. coli* O157:H7, and the main concern in presence of this organism is the possible development of the hemolytic-uremic syndrome. None of the other complications is likely to be associated with this type of *E. coli*. (NMS M&ID, 3rd Ed. p. 67, 144–5, 457)

60. The answer is C. *Shigella dysenteriae* Type 1 re-leases Shiga toxin, a cytotoxin that kills Vero cells and causes the hemolytic-uremic syndrome. Because of the

similar characteristics between this toxin and the one re-leased by *E. coli* O157:H7, the latter is often referred to as "Shiga-like toxin." None of the other listed bacteria have been shown to produce this toxin. (NMS M&ID, 3rd Ed. p. 145, 147)

61. The answer is B. This patient is most likely suffer-ing from a bacterial pneumonia caused by *S. pneumo-niae*. Older individuals are at a higher risk for this infec-tion and are one of the groups for which immunization has been strongly advised. None of the other listed ap-proaches is very practical, for different reasons. There may be no better way to treat his kidney insufficiency than the one that is being followed (not enough informa-tion to judge), and even the best treatment would not change the fact that he is predisposed to contract pneu-mococcal infections, just on the basis of age. Isolation is impractical, there is no easy way to know who is in-fected. Administration of gamma globulin may work, but is expensive and should be reserved for immuno-compromised individuals, known not to respond to im-munization with the pneumococcal vaccine. Prophylac-tic administration of penicillin presents problems of compliance, and in addition, more and more isolates of *S. pneumoniae* are resistant to penicillin. (NMS M&ID, 3rd Ed. p. 95, 110–2, 420–1)

62. The answer is C. The clinical picture is characteris-tic of tetanus, which is caused by *Clostridium tetani*. The clinical symptoms of tetanus are caused by the release of tetanospasmin, a potent neurotoxin that in-hibits the release of neurologic inhibitory transmitters. Thus, muscle contractions are exaggerated in time and intensity, taking the appearance of spasms or contrac-tures. Other clostridia have toxins with effects listed as choices: the α-toxin of *C. perfringens* is a lecithinase, able to hydrolyze lecithin and sphingomyelin-containing phospholipids; botulin, released by *C. botulinum* inter-feres with the release of acetylcholine at the neuromus-cular junctions. (NMS M&ID, 3rd Ed. p. 118–23)

63. The answer is E. *Clostridium* and *Bacillus* are the only two spore-forming genera of medically important bacteria. Both species are gram-positive, but *Clostrid-ium* is anaerobic and *Bacillus* is aerobic. (NMS M&ID, 3rd Ed. p. 118–24)

64. The answer is A. Perioral abscesses after dental ex-traction are often caused by anaerobic organisms com-monly found in the gingival sulcus. Of the listed genera, *Actinomyces, Mycobacterium, Nocardia,* and *Strepto-myces* would fit into the descriptor of "branching, fila-mentous," but *Mycobacterium* and *Nocardia* stain faintly (if at all) with the Gram stain and are usually identified by their staining with acid-fast dyes. *Strepto-myces* is gram-positive, but is a soil organism, aerobic, and usually causes subcutaneous infections in the lower limbs. (NMS M&ID, 3rd Ed. p. 189–91).

65. The answer is C. Methicillin is a penicillinase-resistant, semisynthetic penicillin. The mechanism by which *Staphylococcus aureus* has developed resistance to this antibiotic has been the selection of mutant strains with altered penicillin-binding proteins that retain their enzymatic activity (essential for bacterial growth) but have considerably reduced affinity for β-lactam antibiotics. (NMS M&ID, 3rd Ed. p. 54–7).

66. The answer is C. *H. influenzae* type B is a strictly human pathogen, always transmitted from person to person. Although most strains of *E. coli* are transmitted from person to person, *E. coli* O157:H7 is a zoonotic organism that is acquired from contaminated food products. All other bacteria listed as possible choices have animal reservoirs. (NMS M&ID, 3rd Ed. p. 116–7, 135, 144–5, 148–50, 155).

67. The answer is A. Although several of the mechanisms listed may contribute to the onset of disseminated intravascular coagulation (DIC), disseminated endothelial damage is the common denominator that triggers DIC, whether it is caused by direct infection of endothelial cells, or as a consequence of macrophage activation and overexpression of cell adhesion molecules, which leads to cytotoxic damage of the endothelium. Direct or indirect (complement-mediated) activation of the clotting system is a second major contributor, and endotoxin release could play the key role in macrophage activation. (NMS M&ID, 3rd Ed. p. 68–70, 412–3).

68. The answer is C. The association of kidney stones with infection with a gram-negative rod and alkaline urine are highly suggestive of *Proteus* infection. Bacteria of the genus *Proteus* produce urease and split urea-forming ammonia, which raises the urine pH and causes the precipitation of magnesium phosphate and other salts, creating kidney stones (NMS M&ID, 3rd Ed. p. 160, 451).

69. The answer is E. *Proteus* species are highly motile and their colonies are characteristically described as "swarming." *E. coli* strains isolated from the urinary tract are often hemolytic. *Pseudomonas* and *Klebsiella* colonies can be described as mucoid, and cultures of *Pseudomonas* can be pigmented because of the release of pyocyanin and pyoverdin, although these pigments usually diffuse into the agar. Prodigiosin-producing *Serratia* colonies are bright red. (NMS M&ID, 3rd Ed. p. 144–5, 159–62).

70. The answer is B. Group B *Streptococcus* and *E. coli,* followed by *Listeria monocytogenes,* are the most common agents involved in early neonatal infections. Both *E. coli* and *Moraxella* are gram-negative organisms. The other listed characteristics are typical of group B *Streptococcus*. *Streptococcus pyogenes* is bacitracin-sensitive and *Staphylococci* are catalase-positive.(NMS M&ID, 3rd Ed. p. 105–10, 429–34).

71. The answer is E. At this time, the favored hypothesis is the synthesis of cross-reactive antibodies that react with glomerular antigens. Other proposed pathogenic mechanisms, such as the deposition of preformed immune complexes or the formation of immune complexes in situ, involving streptococcal antigens fixed by glomerular tissues and circulating antistreptococcal antibodies, have not been supported by the available evidence. (NMS M&ID, 3rd Ed. p. 107).

72. The answer is C. M protein, with its antiphagocytic and anticomplement activities, is the major virulence factor for Group A *Streptococcus* and, therefore, its production closely correlates with the pathogenicity of this organism. All other listed factors have some pathogenic role, but of considerably less significance than M protein. (NMS M&ID, 3rd Ed. p. 107).

73. The answer is B. These organisms have in common the fact that their portal of entry are mucosal surfaces, which are rich in IgA antibodies; production of IgA proteases is a common virulence mechanism, affording some degree of protection against the neutralizing effects of these antibodies. While *N. gonorrhoeae* and *H. influenzae* often produce β-lactamases, such is not the case for *N. meningitidis* and *S. pneumoniae*. Lipopolysaccharide (endotoxin) in only found in gram-negative organisms (*S. pneumoniae* is gram-positive). Protein A is exclusive of *Staphylococcus aureus* and protein G of group A *Streptococcus*. (NMS M&ID, 3rd Ed. p. 102–3, 107, 110–2, 126, 133–5).

74. The answer is A. The most likely explanation is that the *lac*+ and pen^R bacteria carried two plasmids, one which included the transfer factor, and the other which did not, but was mobilized by the first. The efficiency of transmission would be better for the plasmid carrying the transfer factor, which should be the one coding for pen^R. All other explanations are implausible. If the transfer of the two traits was independent, either by transformation or by transduction, the transmission of the two traits should happen in similar rates, and it would not be likely that all recipient bacteria that received genetic material acquired one trait and only half acquired the other. Hfr recombination can be ruled out because the recipient bacteria do not usually become conjugation-dependent, therefore they would not likely transfer their newly acquired traits to other bacteria. (NMS M&ID, 3rd Ed. p. 28–34).

75. The answer is E. All components listed are either unique to gram-negative bacteria, or, as in the case of peptidoglycan and polysaccharide capsules, shared by both gram-positive and gram-negative bacteria (NMS M&ID, 3rd Ed. p. 7–12).

76. The answer is C. The acellular pertussis vaccine is a mixture (or recombinant) of inactive toxin and one or several proteins that serve as adhesion factors. The vaccine is more immunogenic and safer than the classic killed bacteria vaccine. (NMS M&ID, 3rd Ed. p. 84–5).

77. The answer is D. The case scenario is that of a bacterial pneumonia caused by an organism that can be identified as *H. influenzae* by its morphological and cultural characteristics. The currently used and highly effective vaccines against this organism are conjugates of capsular polysaccharide with a bacterial toxoid or some other immunogenic protein. (NMS M&ID, 3rd Ed. p. 84–5).

78. The answer is A. The clinical scenario is suggestive of an infection acquired by inoculation of the infectious agent on a region that drains to the axillary lymph nodes. The identification of *Bartonella henselae* allows the physician to establish a diagnosis of cat scratch disease. (NMS M&ID, 3rd Ed. p. 201–2).

79. The answer is G. *Legionella pneumophila* should come to mind when investigating the cause of pneumonia associated with diarrhea occurring in an old veteran with chronic bronchitis. Legionella is difficult to visualize by the Gram stain and does not grow in conventional media, but can be cultured on charcoal-yeast agar supplemented with cysteine (NMS M&ID, 3rd Ed. p. 185–7).

80. The answer is A. The radiograph shows an interstitial pneumonia, which can be caused by a variety of bacteria, viruses, and fungi, but the positive cold agglutinin disease is strongly suggestive of an infection by *Mycoplasma pneumoniae,* which characteristically affects adolescents and young adults and is associated with nonproductive cough and bilateral signs of infiltration. β-lactam antibodies, which interfere with peptidoglycan cross-linking, are not effective against *M. pneumoniae,* which lacks a cell wall. (NMS M&ID, 3rd Ed. p. 187–9)

81. The answer is D. Intra-abdominal abscesses are usually caused by contamination with intestinal bacteria, part of the individual's normal flora. The intestinal normal flora included gram-positive and gram-negative organisms, aerobes and anaerobes, and there is always a good possibility that these bacteria may be resistant to some of the most commonly used antibiotics. What is not likely is that they would secrete enterotoxins, be-

cause those bacteria cause acute gastroenteritis and are eliminated from the intestinal flora. (NMS M&ID, 3rd Ed. p. 100, 469–70)

82. The answer is D. Botulism—the disease caused by ingestion of botulin, the neurotoxin released by *Clostridium botulinum*—is characterized by descending paralysis, which affects initially the cranial nerves (diplopia, dysphagia), progressing centripetally to other nerves (paralytic ileum, urinary retention), and eventually to respiratory paralysis and death. Diarrhea does not occur in this form of food poisoning. (NMS M&ID, 3rd Ed. p. 120–1)

83. The answer is C. In general terms, linkage between 2 bacterial genes is established by determining if they are frequently co-transferred by any of the processes used by bacteria to transfer chromosomal material among themselves, i.e., Hfr conjugation, transduction, and transformation. However, for this approach to work, it is essential that the transfer involves sufficiently large pieces of DNA to contain both genes, if indeed they are linked. This could be associated with generalized transduction, when the phage capsid encloses a relatively large piece of bacterial chromosome, but it is not possible in the case of specialized transduction, which results in the transfer of a very small piece of DNA from either one of the regions flanking the insertion points of a prophage. (NMS M&ID, 3rd Ed. p. 28–34)

84. The answer is D. The lipopolysaccharide of gram-negative bacteria is a structural component of all bacteria in the group, and its synthesis is independent of the presence or absence of plasmids. As a rule, plasmid-coded compounds are not present in all members of a species and account for differences in virulence between isolates. This general characteristic applies to antibiotic resistance, expression of adhesion factors, and synthesis of enterotoxins (all are often coded by plasmid genes) and conjugating ability (always coded by a plasmid gene, even if integrated). (NMS M&ID, 3rd Ed. p. 34–5, 65–70)

85. The answer is D. The main problem in this scenario is administering a live, attenuated vaccine that may be followed by transmission to the immunocompromised sibling and cause severe disease, possibly fatal. Of the attenuated vaccines, the oral polio vaccine is the most dangerous because the virus is shed in the feces, while attenuated vaccines administered by inoculation (such as measles-mumps-rubella), which are not shed by the recipient, are considerably less likely to be transmitted from person to person. The other three vaccines are not live vaccines and have no special risk in an immunocompromised individual. (NMS M&ID, 3rd Ed. p.84; IMI 4th Ed., p. 232–4).

TEST 3

Virology

Test 3

Virology

LIST OF COMMON ABBREVIATIONS

ARDS	adult respiratory distress syndrome
CMV	cytomegalovirus
CNS	central nervous system
CSF	cerebrospinal fluid
DNA	deoxyribonucleic acid
EBV	Epstein-Barr virus
HB_cAg	hepatitis B c antigen
HB_eAg	hepatitis B e antigen
HB_sAg	hepatitis B surface antigen

HBIG	hepatitis B immune globulin
HBV	hepatitis B virus
HIV	human immunodeficiency virus
HSV	herpes simplex virus
HTLV-1	human T-cell lymphoma/leukemia virus
ICAM-1	intercellular adhesion molecule-1
Ig	immunoglobulin
LFA	lymphocyte function associated antigen
MHC	major histocompatibility complex
RNA	ribonucleic acid

LIST OF BACTERIA

E. coli *Escherichia coli*
S. aureus *Staphylococcus aureus*

DIRECTIONS: (Items 1–56) Each of the numbered items or incomplete statements in this section is followed by answers or by completions of the statement. Select the ONE lettered answer or completion that is BEST in each case.

1. A murine leukemia virus is best defined by which combinations of characteristics below?

	Genome	Oncogene	Transmission	Oncogenic potential
(A)	Complete	None	Horizontal, vertical	Low
(B)	Complete	None	Horizontal, vertical	High
(C)	Complete	Present	Horizontal, vertical	High
(D)	Incomplete	Present	Horizontal, vertical	Low
(E)	Incomplete	Present	Vertical	High

QUESTIONS 2–4

A 32-year-old female HBV carrier with a history of intravenous drug abuse seeks medical attention because she has become pregnant. In evaluating the risk of infection to the fetus, you run a battery of serological tests.

2. Which of the following tests is most indicative of high infectivity when positive?

(A) HB_sAg
(B) HB_cAg
(C) HB_eAg
(D) Anti-HB_sAg
(E) Anti-HB_eAg

3. In trying to assess interventions that could possibly reduce the risk of infection to the baby, which one of these infection routes is most frequently involved in the vertical transmission of HBV?

(A) Fetal contact with infected blood during childbirth
(B) Ingestion of the virus present in maternal breast milk
(C) Transplacental transmission of the virus

4. Which measure should be taken to prevent fetal infection?

(A) Administer HBIG to the baby at birth
(B) Immunize the mother during pregnancy and administer HBIG to the baby at birth
(C) Immunize the mother during pregnancy and immunize the neonate with a first dose administered at birth
(D) Immunize the neonate with a first dose administered at birth
(E) Simultaneously administer, at different sites, HBIG and hepatitis B vaccine to the baby at birth

5. The association of neoplastic transformation with p53 mutations is a result of the altered ability of mutated p53 protein to

(A) Activate membrane-associated G proteins
(B) Phosphorylate tyrosine-containing substrates
(C) Promote DNA repair
(D) Stimulate entry into the M phase of the cell cycle
(E) Transduce signals from growth factor receptors

6. A retrovirus is found in a high proportion of laboratory mice. Most viremic animals are asymptomatic, but others develop a fatal wasting syndrome, and a few develop leukemia and other tumors after long periods of latency. The virus in question most likely lacks the following gene

(A) *Gag*
(B) *Pol*
(C) *Env*
(D) *Onc*

7. Which of the following viruses can interfere with hematopoiesis by infecting undifferentiated stem cells?

(A) Ebola virus
(B) EBV
(C) HTLV-1
(D) JC virus
(E) Parvovirus B 19

8. The avian flu outbreak in Hong Kong at the end of 1997 was believed to be caused by

(A) A new strain emerging from reassortment of human and avian viruses
(B) The emergence of a new human strain by antigenic drift of an avian virus
(C) Human infection by an avian virus that previously had not crossed the species barrier
(D) The spontaneous appearance of a new influenza virus strain that infects both humans and birds with equal effectiveness
(E) The feeding of poultry with antimicrobial agents that facilitated the emergence of new viral strains

9. The vaccine currently used to prevent hepatitis B infections is constituted by

(A) Conjugate of HB$_s$Ag and a bacterial toxoid
(B) HB$_s$Ag isolated from chronic carriers
(C) Inactivated HBV
(D) Recombinant HB$_s$Ag
(E) Recombinant vaccinia virus expressing HB$_s$Ag

QUESTIONS 10–11

A 4-month-old child is brought to the emergency room in respiratory distress. Physical examination shows a mildly cyanotic infant with diffuse rhonchi and rales on lung auscultation. The radiograph is suggestive of bilateral bronchopneumonia. A nasopharyngeal swab was sent for culture and direct examination. The initial cultures were negative, but the pathologist reports finding large multinucleated cellular clumps in the swab.

10. This infection is most likely caused by

(A) CMV
(B) EBV
(C) HSV
(D) Human herpesvirus 6
(E) Respiratory syncytial virus

11. The antiviral agent best suited for treating this child is

(A) Acyclovir
(B) Amantadine
(C) Ganciclovir
(D) Ribavirin
(E) Vidarabine

QUESTIONS 12–14

A child presents with multiple vesicular eruptions on the mucous membranes of the mouth, which resolve spontaneously within 3 weeks. However, during the next 12 months, the child suffers several recurrent infections, characterized by blisters in the epidermomucosal junction of the perioral region. In all cases there is complete spontaneous recovery followed by symptom-free intervals.

12. This is a manifestation of an infection best described as

(A) Latent
(B) Lytic
(C) Persistent
(D) Subclinical
(E) Transforming

13. The child's symptoms will most likely be alleviated with

(A) A blocker of nucleic acid release
(B) A reverse transcriptase inhibitor
(C) A viral protease inhibitor
(D) An activator of cellular ribonucleases
(E) An inhibitor of viral DNA synthesis

14. The low toxicity of the antiviral agents used to treat this infection is a consequence of the fact that these drugs

- (A) Block a viral enzyme that has no homologue in human cells
- (B) Block specifically the penetration and uncoating of the viral nucleic acid
- (C) Inhibit the activity of a viral protease that processes viral proteins but has no effect on human proteins
- (D) Only become active after a series of phosphorylations initiated by a viral thymidine kinase
- (E) Penetrate noninfected cells very poorly

QUESTIONS 15–17

A 24-year-old medical student is admitted to a tertiary hospital with headaches, fever, and nuchal rigidity. A computed tomography scan of the head is normal and CSF examination shows mild leukocytosis with lymphocyte predominance. Agglutination tests and cultures for agents known to cause meningitis are negative. A tuberculin test is negative.

15. This situation is most likely being caused by

- (A) Arboviruses
- (B) Enteroviruses
- (C) HSV
- (D) Paramyxoviruses
- (E) Retroviruses

16. The agent in question was most likely acquired by

- (A) Ingestion
- (B) Inhalation
- (C) Inoculation by a vector
- (D) Intravenous injection
- (E) Sexual contact

17. An *S. aureus* broth culture is infected with a large number of copies of a phenotypically mixed bacteriophage with nucleic acid type 128, obtained from an *E. coli*-infecting phage, and protein coat type 135, specific for an *S. aureus*-infecting phage. To recover the phage progeny from this culture, the ultrafiltrate of the broth should be added to a second culture of

- (A) *E. coli*
- (B) *S. aureus*
- (C) Either organism

18. A virus is added to two cell lines—A and B. After 30 minutes no infective particles can be recovered from either cell line. After 12 hours, infective particles can be recovered from the culture medium of cell line A but not from the culture medium of cell line B. The monolayer of cell line B appears undisturbed and is checked again at 24 hours, but infective particles continue to be absent in the culture medium. The most likely explanation for these findings is that cell line B

- (A) Does not allow penetration of the virus
- (B) Does not express transacting proteins that promote viral gene expression
- (C) Is persistently infected by the virus with minimal adverse effects
- (D) Is rapidly lysed by the virus, before it can complete its replication cycle
- (E) Lacks receptors for the virus

19. Which of the following is an important general characteristic of the replication of (−)RNA viruses?

- (A) Genomic migration to the nucleus
- (B) Release from infected cells by cell lysis
- (C) Requirement of an RNA-dependent RNA polymerase packed in the virion
- (D) Structural proteins derive from postsynthetically spliced polyproteins

20. Which of the following diseases is usually spread by respiratory secretions?

- (A) ARDS associated with the Sin Nombre virus
- (B) Dengue
- (C) Measles
- (D) Viral encephalitis
- (E) Yellow fever

QUESTIONS 21–22

An outbreak of viral encephalitis is detected in Ocala, Florida. Blood is obtained from 6 affected individuals and complement fixation tests are run to detect antibodies against the most common arboviruses in the Eastern United States. The results of the tests are shown in the table.

Arbovirus	Subject A	Subject B	Subject C	Subject D	Subject E
Eastern equine encephalitis	10/20*	<10/<10	40/40	20/<40	20/20
St. Louis encephalitis	<10/<10	<10/<10	10/<10	<10/10	<10/<10
Western equine encephalitis	20/160	40/160	10/1	10/320	20/80
Venezuelan encephalitis	160/160	10/10	<10/10	40/20	80/160

*Results expressed as acute titer/convalescent titer

21. Which of the listed arboviruses does not appear to be prevalent in Ocala?

(A) Eastern equine encephalitis virus
(B) St. Louis encephalitis
(C) Venezuelan encephalitis
(D) Western equine encephalitis

22. The most likely vector to have transmitted the infectious agent involved in this outbreak is the

(A) Flea
(B) Horse fly
(C) Mosquito
(D) Sand fly
(E) Tick

23. Among the early proteins coded in the adenovirus genome, there are proteins able to

(A) Code for capsid proteins
(B) Induce hyperexpression of MHC-I molecules on the cell membrane
(C) Inhibit the function of p53
(D) Initiate the viral genome transcription
(E) Phosphorylate ganciclovir

QUESTIONS 24–25

A young, unmarried woman in her second month of pregnancy is found to be HIV-positive on an enzyme immunoassay. She denies intravenous drug use. She is not certain about the HIV status of the father, who has recently left the area, and did not use safe sex practices. The patient's serum was sent to a reference laboratory for Western blot.

24. Of the following diagrams reproducing results of Western blots for HIV antibodies, which one is most likely to correspond to this patient?

25. To significantly reduce the risk of maternofetal transmission of HIV infection, it is recommended to give zidovudine to the

(A) Mother during delivery and to the newborn for 6 weeks
(B) Mother from week 14 until birth
(C) Mother from week 14 until birth and to the newborn for 6 weeks
(D) Mother from week 14 until labor
(E) Newborn for 6 weeks

26. Hemagglutination-inhibition is used to obtain serological evidence of infection caused by

(A) Adenovirus
(B) CMV
(C) EBV
(D) Influenza A
(E) Measles

27. The transmission of Hantaviruses usually requires exposure to

(A) Contaminated airborne droplets
(B) Contaminated water
(C) Mosquitoes
(D) Ticks
(E) Rodent excreta

28. Which of the following viruses is most likely to use the human intestinal mucosa as its portal of entry?

(A) A naked (−)RNA virus
(B) A naked (+)RNA virus
(C) An enveloped (+)RNA virus
(D) An enveloped DNA virus
(E) An enveloped virus with affinity to mucosal cells

29. Which of the following diseases caused by viruses can be prevented in experimental animals by administering immunosuppressive drugs?

(A) Acute murine leukemia
(B) Lymphocytic choriomeningitis
(C) Sarcoma
(D) Scrapie
(E) Viral encephalitis

30. Which ONE of the following characteristics is common to the products of most transforming genes found in DNA tumor virus?

(A) Ability to inactivate tumor suppressor gene products
(B) Ability to induce intracellular signal cascades
(C) Ability to induce the expression of genes controlling cell proliferation
(D) Induction as a consequence of chromosomal translocations
(E) Nuclear binding proteins that can induce cell division

31. A 27-year-old white man was brought to the hospital by emergency personnel. His complaints included fever (104°F, 40°C), chills, headache, backache, and nausea. There was evidence of vomit on his clothing. A workup by the resident revealed that he recently participated in a Peace Corps project in Puerto Cabello, Venezuela. After admission, gastric endoscopy revealed hemorrhagic areas of the stomach, small intestine, and colon. His direct serum bilirubin level was 5 mg/dL. His arterial blood pressure was 100/60. Which of the following measures could have most effectively protected this young man against the disease he contracted?

(A) Avoidance of uncooked shellfish
(B) Avoidance of unsafe water and fresh vegetables
(C) Inoculation with an attenuated virus
(D) Prophylactic administration of ribavirin
(E) Use of a mosquito net at bedtime

32. Which of the following viruses reaches its target organ by hematogenous dissemination?

(A) HSV
(B) Papillomavirus
(C) Rhinovirus
(D) Rotavirus
(E) Rubella virus

33. Protection against influenza A virus in a nonimmune individual can be achieved by administering a drug that interferes with

(A) Activity of the viral endonuclease
(B) Binding of host mRNA caps by the viral P1 protein
(C) Synthesis of viral progeny RNA
(D) Uncoating of viral nucleic acid
(E) Viral adsorption and penetration

34. Prophylaxis against the common cold can be achieved by administering an aerosol containing the following compound

(A) Monoclonal anti-Rhinovirus antibody
(B) Recombinant CR2
(C) Recombinant ICAM-1
(D) Recombinant LFA-1
(E) Recombinant rhinovirus capsid proteins

35. Which of the following is an important characteristic of the replication of naked (+)RNA viruses?

(A) Integration in the host genome
(B) Release from infected cells by budding
(C) Replication in the nucleus
(D) Requirement for an RNA-dependent RNA polymerase packed in the virion
(E) Structural proteins derive from postsynthetically spliced polyproteins

36. A major biological advantage of the attenuated poliovirus vaccine relative to the inactivated vaccine is its

(A) Ability to immunize simultaneously against the major types of poliovirus
(B) Ability to induce circulating antibodies of all isotypes
(C) Greater safety
(D) Induction of mucosal immunity
(E) Propagation to close contacts of immunized children

37. Acute leukemia viruses induce malignant transformation by

    (A) Activation of a cellular oncogene as a consequence of LTR integration
    (B) Infection by a replication-competent retrovirus
    (C) Insertion on the host cell genome of an actively expressed transforming oncogene
    (D) Postinsertional chromosomal translocations leading to the activation of *c-myc*
    (E) Synthesis of viral proteins that inactivate tumor suppressor gene products of the host cell

38. Laryngotracheobronchitis (croup) in children is most often caused by

    (A) Adenoviruses
    (B) Influenza viruses
    (C) Parainfluenza virus type 1
    (D) Respiratory syncytial virus
    (E) Rhinoviruses

39. The virus that causes the production of heterophile antibodies capable of agglutinating horse erythrocytes is

    (A) Adenovirus
    (B) CMV
    (C) EBV
    (D) Influenza A
    (E) Measles

40. Which of the following transforming genes modifies NFkB and causes the overexpression of interleukin and interleukin–receptor-coding genes?

    (A) Adenovirus E1A gene product
    (B) Burkitt's lymphoma *myc* gene product
    (C) HIV *tat* gene product
    (D) HTLV-1 *tax* gene product
    (E) Polyoma virus T antigen

QUESTIONS 41–42

A 7-year-old patient receiving chemotherapy for acute lymphocytic leukemia develops a generalized vesicular eruption associated with fever and malaise. An acute and a convalescent serum sample was sent for viral antibody studies with the following results

	Acute Serum	Convalescent Serum
Herpes simplex	1:16	1:8
Human herpesvirus 6	1:8	1:8
Varicella-zoster	1:8	1:32
Coxsackie A-16	1:8	1:16

41. This is most likely a case of

    (A) Atypical Coxsackie A-16 infection
    (B) Chickenpox
    (C) Herpes
    (D) Roseola infantum
    (E) Shingles

42. In immunocompetent individuals, this disease can be prevented by administering

    (A) A mixed component vaccine
    (B) A recombinant vaccine
    (C) An attenuated vaccine
    (D) An inactivated vaccine
    (E) Immune γ-globulin

43. The virus most likely to pack an RNA-dependent RNA polymerase in its virions is

    (A) HBV
    (B) HSV
    (C) HIV
    (D) Poliovirus
    (E) Respiratory syncytial virus

44. Which characteristics best apply to the viral agent that causes progressive multifocal leukoencephalopathy?

    (A) (+)RNA virus that has special affinity for microglial cells
    (B) Defective particles that evade the immune system and cause persistent infection of neural cells
    (C) Enveloped DNA virus that latently infects neural cells and is reactivated under stressful conditions
    (D) Latent DNA virus that causes clinical infection in immunocompromised patients
    (E) Unconventional agent that causes a spongiform encephalopathy

45. Which mode of transmission is characteristic of a (+)RNA naked virus that causes jaundice in temperate regions?

    (A) Inhalation of aerosolized secretions
    (B) Blood transfusion
    (C) Sexual intercourse
    (D) Ingestion of contaminated food or water
    (E) Mosquito bites

46. Cells transformed in culture by oncogenic viruses characteristically have which property?

(A) Decreased agglutinability by lectins
(B) Decreased survival
(C) Increased rate of glucose transport across the cell membrane
(D) Increased expression of MHC molecules
(E) Increased serum requirements

47. Herpesvirus resistance to acyclovir is usually observed in association with

(A) Abnormally active cellular nucleotide kinases
(B) Decreased synthesis of transport-associated proteins
(C) Mutation of the viral DNA polymerase
(D) Synthesis of an inactivating protein
(E) Thymidine kinase deficiency

48. Which of the following cellular effects of type I interferons (α and β) is believed to play a key role in antiviral protection?

(A) Down-regulation of the expression of viral receptors on the cell membrane
(B) Induction of an adenine nucleotide with RNAse activity
(C) Inhibition of viral polymerases
(D) Inhibition of viral proteases
(E) Interference with viral nucleic acid release in the cytoplasm

49. Which one of the following techniques can indicate whether infective viral particles are present in a sample?

(A) Detection of viral antigens by enzyme immunoassay
(B) Direct immunofluorescence with labeled antibodies
(C) Hemadsorption
(D) Polymerase chain reaction amplification of viral genomic sequences
(E) Plaque formation assay

50. The host's immune response is most likely to play a significant pathogenic role in

(A) Chronic viral hepatitis
(B) Fulminant viral hepatitis
(C) Paralytic poliomyelitis
(D) Viral meningitis
(E) Warts

51. The mother of an 18-month-old girl seeks medical attention because her daughter is febrile, restless, and refuses food. Physical examination is unremarkable except that several small vesicular lesions, some ulcerated, are seen in the tonsils and posterior pharynx. The agent most likely to cause this disease is a

(A) (+)RNA enterovirus
(B) (−)RNA paramyxovirus
(C) Double-stranded (ds) DNA herpesvirus
(D) dsDNA poxvirus
(E) Single-stranded (ss)DNA parvovirus

52. The T antigen of SV40 and the early gene products of adenoviruses and papilloma viruses can

(A) Activate a membrane-associated protein kinase
(B) Activate proteins controlling the cell division cycle
(C) Bind to NFkB
(D) Inactivate p53
(E) Inhibit the transport of MHC-peptide complexes to the cell membrane

53. Comparing the two available polio vaccines, a unique biological property of the oral poliovirus vaccine is that it

(A) Induces a systemic IgA response
(B) Induces hemagglutination-inhibiting antibodies
(C) Induces IgG neutralizing antibodies
(D) Prevents the dissemination of poliovirus to the nervous system
(E) Spreads to nonimmunized individuals

54. Which of the following clinical syndromes is associated with the Sin Nombre (*Four Corners*) strain of Hantavirus?

(A) Acute kidney failure
(B) Acute respiratory failure
(C) Hemorrhagic fever
(D) Influenza-like syndrome
(E) Meningitis

55. When human cells in culture are infected by HSV type 1, viral nucleic acid replication begins at 6 hours after infection. Gene A codes for the viral DNA polymerase and gene B codes for a capsid protein. If acyclovir is added to the cell culture at the same time as the virus, which of the following patterns of detection is likely to be observed?

	Viral DNA polymerase	Capsid protein
(A)	Detectable at 4 hours	Not detectable at any time
(B)	Detectable at 4 hours	Detectable at 10 hours
(C)	Detectable at 10 hours	Detectable at 10 hours
(D)	Not detectable at any time	Detectable at 10 hours
(E)	Not detectable at any time	Not detectable at any time

56. A 32-year-old Colombian businessman who has just arrived in Miami from Cartagena checks into the emergency room of the University of Miami Hospital complaining of fever, intense headaches, and excruciating pain in the joint and muscular masses of the upper and lower limbs. His vital signs are:

Temperature: 104°F (40°C)
Respiration: 32 per minute
Blood pressure (sitting): 130/80
On physical examination, a faint macular rash in the trunk is noted. Remaining examination is within normal limits, including the neurologic examination. Until proven otherwise, this patent should be considered as having contracted

(A) Dengue
(B) Machupo virus hemorrhagic fever
(C) Viral encephalitis
(D) Viral influenza
(E) Yellow fever

Directions: (Items 57–60) Each of the numbered items or incomplete statements in this section is negatively phrased, as indicated by a capitalized word such as NOT, LEAST, or EXCEPT. Select the ONE lettered answer or completion that is BEST suited in each case.

57. In a cell culture, if a drug able to block DNA synthesis (such as actinomycin D) is added at the time of infection, which of the following viruses will NOT replicate?

(A) Bunyaviruses
(B) Echoviruses
(C) Hepatitis virus E
(D) Herpes viruses
(E) Reoviruses

58. When a susceptible cell line is infected with adenovirus type 2 in the presence of adenine arabinoside (Ara-A, vidarabine), which of the following viral components will NOT be synthesized?

(A) Capsid proteins
(B) DNA polymerase
(C) DNA-binding protein
(D) Transactivating proteins
(E) MHC-binding protein (gp19)

59. Five different viruses were added to cell cultures pre-treated with actinomycin D, a drug which blocks DNA synthesis. Which of the viruses will NOT generate infectious progeny?

(A) EBV
(B) Hepatitis virus A
(C) Influenza virus type A
(D) Poliovirus type III
(E) Yellow fever virus

60. Of the following diseases with cutaneous expression, all are caused by a virus from the human herpesvirus family EXCEPT

(A) Chickenpox
(B) Infectious mononucleosis
(C) Kaposi's sarcoma
(D) Molluscum contagiosum
(E) Roseola infantum

ANSWER KEY

1. A	13. E	25. C	37. C	49. E
2. C	14. D	26. D	38. C	50. A
3. A	15. B	27. E	39. C	51. A
4. E	16. A	28. B	40. D	52. D
5. C	17. A	29. B	41. B	53. E
6. D	18. B	30. A	42. C	54. B
7. E	19. C	31. C	43. E	55. A
8. C	20. C	32. E	44. D	56. A
9. D	21. B	33. D	45. D	57. D
10. E	22. C	34. C	46. C	58. A
11. D	23. C	35. E	47. E	59. A
12. A	24. B	36. D	48. B	60. D

ANSWERS AND EXPLANATIONS

Note: Page numbers designated as "IMI 4th Ed" refer to *Introduction to Medical Immunology,* 4th ed., New York/Basel, Marcel Dekker, 1998. Page numbers designated as "NMS M&ID 3rd Ed" refer to *NMS Microbiology and Infectious Diseases,* 3rd ed. Baltimore, Williams & Wilkins, 1997. Page numbers indicated as "PAInfDis 4th Ed" refer to Reese RE, Betts RF, eds., *Practical Approach to Infectious Diseases,* 4th ed., Boston, Little, Brown & Co., 1996.

1. The answer is A. The animal leukemia viruses have been extensively studied and are the best characterized models of oncoviruses, on which most of our knowledge about these viruses is based. Structurally, the animal leukemia viruses are nondefective retroviruses that do not contain an oncogene in their genome and cause malignancies sporadically, due to insertional mutagenesis. In contrast, the acute leukemia viruses carry active oncogenes in their genomes and cause leukemias and sarcomas with high frequency. Most of the viruses of this last group have incomplete genomes; that is, when they acquired the oncogene, they lost one or more than one of the structural genes and their replication depends on co-infection with closely related viruses. One exception is the Rous sarcoma virus, which has a complete, infective genome, including an oncovirus. (NMS M&ID, 3rd Ed. p. 257–9)

2. The answer is C. All HBV carriers, by definition, are positive in tests for the Hb$_s$Ag. Those that are also positive for the HB$_e$Ag are considered more infectious. This is because the HB$_e$Ag derives from the HB$_c$ Ag (which remains intracellular) and its presence means that more than a single layer of viral proteins is expressed in infected cells. Therefore, the likelihood of having full infectious particles in circulation is increased. The detection of antibodies, in contrast, is indicative of a strong immune response against the virus and is associated with a lower degree of infectivity. (NMS M&ID, 3rd Ed. p. 324–7)

3. The answer is A. The most usual mechanism of transmission of HBV to a neonate is perinatal exposure to blood and body fluids from an infected mother. More rarely, the virus can be transmitted transplacentally or via breast milk. (NMS M&ID, 3rd Ed. p. 482)

4. The answer is E. Neonates born to HBV-infected mothers or to mothers of unknown HBV status should receive both the recombinant vaccine and HBIG within 12 hours of delivery. The combined administration of vaccine and HBIG is 90% protective. It follows that all pregnant women should be tested for HBV infection as part of their routine prenatal care. (NMS M&ID, 3rd Ed. p. 482; PAInfDis, 4th Ed. p. 83)

5. The answer is C. The protein coded by the p53 gene is a tumor suppressor gene, involved in a sequence of control mechanisms that arrest cell proliferation when a DNA mutation takes place, giving the cell the opportunity to repair the mutation. A p53 mutation that results in the loss of this biological function will have no protective effect against neoplastic mutations, and neoplastic transformation will be more likely to occur. All other listed effects are induced by different oncogenes or transforming genes: the *sis* gene product activates the platelet-derived growth factor receptor, which is associated with a G protein in the cell membrane; *src* codes for a protein kinase with tyrosine affinity; *myc* promotes cellular proliferation; *erb* codes for a truncated version of one of the many receptors that mediates cell activation and which, in this abnormal form, is in a state of autoactivation and induces the corresponding cascade of kinases without need for occupancy. (NMS M&ID, 3rd Ed. p. 258)

6. The answer is D. Many animals being infected and viremic suggests that this is a highly infective virus, with a complete genome (with the *gag, pol,* and *env* genes). The fact that only a few animals develop malignancy suggests that the virus does not carry an oncogene, and that malignant transformation depends on insertional mutagenesis. (NMS M&ID, 3rd Ed. p. 257–8)

7. The answer is E. Parvovirus B 19 can infect precursor cells of the erythroid lineage, which express an antigen (P antigen) that serves as the receptor for the virus. The resulting destruction of red cell precursors is particularly severe in children with sickle cell disease, who may develop aplastic crisis as a consequence of the infection. The Ebola virus causes a form of hemorrhagic fever; EBV infects B cells and is associated with Burkitt's lymphoma; HTLV-1 infects CD4 T cells and causes leukemia; the JC virus infects neural calls and causes progressive multifocal leukoencephalopathy. (NMS M&ID, 3rd Ed. p. 291–2)

8. The answer is C. The new H5N1 strain of influenza virus isolated for the first time in Hong Kong in late 1997 appears to be an avian strain of virus that has become able to infect humans. Feeding poultry with antimicrobials has no effect on the emergence of new viruses. (NMS M&ID, 3rd Ed. p. 305–62)

9. The answer is D. The early hepatitis B vaccines were prepared with HB$_s$Ag isolated from chronic carriers, but later the recombinant vaccine was adopted, because of both increased safety and ease of production in large scale. (NMS M&ID, 3rd Ed. p. 85, 327)

10. The answer is E. Respiratory syncytial virus, like most paramyxoviruses and other viruses, including human herpesviruses (HHV 1 and 2), CMV (HHV 5), and EBV (HHV 4), as well as HIV, can fuse infected and noninfected cells, leading to the formation of large masses of agglomerated cells; these can be described as "multinucleated giant cells" or as "syncytia." Neither HSV nor HHV 6, however, commonly cause pneumonia. (NMS M&ID, 3rd Ed. p. 247, 277–9, 313)

11. The answer is D. Ribavirin has been shown to have activity against respiratory syncytial virus, blocking viral protein synthesis. However, its clinical benefit is controversial. Acyclovir is used to treat herpes simplex infection, amantadine is effective against influenza virus, ganciclovir has been used to treat CMV infections, and vidarabine is effective against herpesviruses and other DNA viruses. (NMS M&ID, 3rd Ed. p. 234–8, 313)

12. The answer is A. The clinical picture is typical of herpes, caused in most cases by HSV type I. HSV causes a latent infection of nerve ganglia and the infection is characterized by spontaneous relapses, triggered by stress, fever, and other ill-defined factors. Lytic infection is a term that applies to the effect of a virus on a cell line, rather than to the biological characteristics of that infection. Persistent infections are characterized by constant viremia, which is not found in patients infected with herpes. Subclinical infections are those without clinical expression, which is not the case in herpes. Transforming infections are those that result in the acquisition of malignant characteristics by the infected cells. (NMS M&ID, 3rd Ed. p. 244–6, 251–2, 277–8)

13. The answer is E. Herpesvirus is a DNA virus, and the most effective agents for its treatment are viral-activated nucleosides, such as acyclovir and famciclovir. These agents stop viral DNA synthesis with minimal toxicity to the infected cell. Of the other choices, two correspond to currently used antiviral agents (reverse transcriptase inhibitors and viral protease inhibitors), but their use is limited to RNA viruses (retroviruses and other viruses sharing some of the replication steps of retroviruses). (NMS M&ID, 3rd Ed. p. 234–8)

14. The answer is D. The activity of nucleoside analogs depends on their conversion into triphosphorylated nucleotides. In the case of acyclovir and famciclovir, the first phosphorylation is carried out by a viral thymidine kinase, and the remaining phosphorylations are done by cellular enzymes, but only after the initial viral-dependent phosphorylation has taken place. This results in very low toxicity for noninfected cells, where the drugs will remain inactive. (NMS M&ID, 3rd Ed. p. 236–7)

15. The answer is B. The clinical picture is one of meningitis, and the viral origin is suggested by the predominance of lymphocytes in the CSF and the negativity of the tests for other agents known to cause meningitis. The enteroviruses are, by far, the most common viral causes of meningitis. Arboviruses and HSV are more frequently involved as causes of encephalitis. Paramyxoviruses, such as measles virus, can cause subacute sclerosing panencephalitis, a chronic, degenerative disease of the CNS. Retroviruses can also infect nervous tissue, but the clinical picture is not one of meningitis. (NMS M&ID, 3rd Ed. p. 293–7, 435, 439, 442–5)

16. The answer is A. The main transmission route for all enteroviruses is fecal–oral. (NMS M&ID, 3rd Ed. p. 293)

17. The answer is A. The progeny's characteristics will be determined by the nucleic acid enclosed in this hypothetical pseudotype. Because the genome is that of an *E. coli*–infecting phage, the progeny will express the surface proteins coded by the genome, which will interact with *E. coli* receptors, but not with *S. aureus* receptors. (NMS M&ID, 3rd Ed. p. 228–9)

18. The answer is B. That the virus is not recoverable 30 minutes after being added to cell line B proves that it reacted with cell receptors and was internalized. The stage in which virus is not detectable from an infected cell line is known as eclipse phase. Three hypotheses remain to possibly explain why viral progeny is not recovered from cell line. Premature death of the infected cells is ruled out because the monolayer remains intact. Persistent infection with minimal cytopathology would result in recovery of infectious particles from the supernatant. The best hypothesis is that the virus did not replicate because the cell line was not suitable. Viral replication often requires the "collaboration" of the infected cells that provide transacting proteins able to activate the expression of viral genes. (NMS M&ID, 3rd Ed. p. 211–3)

19. The answer is C. As a rule all RNA viruses replicate in the cytoplasm (exceptions being the paramyxoviruses and retroviruses) and their release from infected cells varies from species to species (again, as a rule, naked viruses are released by lysis of the infected cell and enveloped viruses are released by budding). The replication of (−)RNA viruses implies one step that cannot be mediated by cellular enzymes, that is, the transcription of (+)RNA strands to be used as a message for the different viral proteins and as templates for viral (−)RNA progeny, and this step is mediated by an RNA–dependent RNA polymerase. That enzyme needs to be packed in the virion, because if it was encoded but not packed, the cellular ribosomes would not be able to translate (−)RNA. As for the processing of polyproteins, that is a characteristic of (+)RNA viruses. (NMS M&ID, 3rd Ed. p. 215–6)

20. The answer is C. Paramyxoviruses, including the measles virus, are spread via contaminated aerosolized respiratory secretions. Dengue, viral encephalitis, and yellow fever are arthropod-borne infections, transmitted by mosquitoes. The Hantavirus known as Sin Nombre is transmitted via contamination of water or food with infected rodent urine. (NMS M&ID, 3rd Ed. p. 299–302, 309–13, 319–20)

21. The answer is B. Looking at the antibody titers, it is obvious that all the tested subjects had not been exposed to St. Louis encephalitis virus. The most likely cause of the outbreak was Western equine encephalitis virus, for which four of the individuals showed fourfold or greater increases in their antibody titer between acute and convalescent samples. (NMS M&ID, 3rd Ed. p. 273–4, 301–2)

22. The answer is C. Several insects can be vectors of a variety of infections, but most arboviruses involved in viral encephalitis (including the Western equine encephalitis virus) are transmitted by mosquitoes both to horses and humans. (NMS M&ID, 3rd Ed. p. 299–302)

23. The answer is C. Among the early proteins encoded in the adenovirus genome there are proteins that inhibit the function of p53 and interfere with MHC-I expression. The initial transcription of the viral genome is carried out by the cellular polymerases and the phosphorylation of ganciclovir is a characteristic of viruses of the herpes group. Capsid proteins, as most structural proteins, are always expressed late in the replication cycle of DNA viruses. (NMS M&ID, 3rd Ed. p. 211–4, 237, 254)

24. The answer is B. A positive Western blot should show antibodies reactive with antigens representative of all major groups—such as envelope glycoproteins (gp160, gp120, and gp41), capsid proteins (p24), the re-

verse transcriptase (p66 and p51), and the viral endonuclease (p31). The Western blots reproduced in the other lanes would be considered indeterminate. (NMS M&ID, 3rd Ed. p. 502–3, 511)

25. The answer is C. Administering zidovudine to the mother from week 14 until and during birth and to the newborn from birth until 6 weeks reduces the 26%–30% frequency of maternal–fetal transmission to 8%. (NMS M&ID, 3rd Ed. p. 511)

26. The answer is D. Orthomyxoviruses, such as influenza A virus, have envelope glycoproteins that react with red cell receptors and cause those cells to agglutinate (viral hemagglutination). The same protein interacts with cellular receptors (membrane sialated glycoproteins) on mucosal epithelium of the upper respiratory tract, which is the portal of entry and main target tissue for influenza virus. Antibodies reacting with the viral hemagglutinin can prevent the infection of susceptible cells in vitro and are also able to prevent viral hemagglutination. Therefore, testing for hemagglutination-inhibiting antibodies is one of the most common serological techniques used to diagnose infections by the influenza virus. (NMS M&ID, 3rd Ed. p. 244, 273, 305–7)

27. The answer is E. Hanta viruses are members of the Bunyavirus family, which includes several genera of arboviruses, but the Hanta viruses are not transmitted by insect vectors. Rather, these viruses infect primarily rodent populations and are excreted on the urine of infected mice. Transmission to humans requires close contact of human and rodent populations. (NMS M&ID, 3rd Ed. p. 319–20)

28. The answer is B. All enveloped viruses are extremely labile because the lipid bilayer that forms the envelope matrix can be easily denatured by a variety of agents. Such viruses, when ingested, will lose infectivity during traffic through the gastrointestinal tract. Naked viruses, in contrast, have a protective coat constituted by protein, which is considerably more resistant to denaturing conditions. Thus, a naked virus is more likely to retain infectivity after ingestion. Note that all (−)RNA viruses pathogenic to humans are enveloped; therefore, choice A, although theoretically correct, is ruled out on the basis that such a virus able to infect humans has yet to be described. (NMS M&ID, 3rd Ed. p. 207–9)

29. The answer is B. Lymphocytic choriomeningitis is caused by an arenavirus that is only mildly cytopathic. The disease is, for the most part, due to the immune response against the virus, as demonstrated by the fact that when neonatal (immunoincompetent) or immunosuppressed mice are infected with this virus, they develop a persistent infection that is considerably less severe than the natural infection on immunocompetent animals. A pathogenic immunologic component is also involved in viral encephalitis, particularly in its secondary forms, but in the case of primary viral encephalitis, the viruses involved are rather pathogenic and administration of immunosuppressive drugs would imply a considerable risk of exacerbating the disease. Immunosuppression is more likely to have adverse effects in animals with viral-induced sarcoma or scrapie. In these diseases, the immune response does not play a pathogenic role. (NMS M&ID, 3rd Ed. p. 249, 266, 319)

30. The answer is A. Most DNA tumor viruses express proteins that inactivate tumor suppressor genes, particularly p53 and the retinoblastoma gene product. Several other choices correspond to the effects of transforming genes unique to a given virus. For example, the EBV expresses two transforming genes—LMP-1 and LMP-2—which can be involved in the activation of intracellular signaling cascades; the adenovirus E1A gene products are transactivating proteins that upregulate cellular genes controlling cell proliferation; and the E2A gene of the same virus encodes a DNA-binding protein that serves as a primer for DNA replication. Chromosomal translocations in Burkitt's lymphoma are associated with overexpression of *c-myc,* but it has not been proven that EBV causes the translocations, and *c-myc* is a cellular proto-oncogene, not a viral-transforming gene. (NMS M&ID, 3rd Ed. p. 217–8, 252–5)

31. The answer is C. The clinical picture is suggestive of a diagnosis of yellow fever: the travel to an endemic area (a coastal, swampy area in Venezuela), the mucosal hemorrhages associated with jaundice, and the decrease in blood pressure are all characteristic of the disease. The most effective prophylactic measure is immunization with an attenuated vaccine, which is recommended for travelers to high-risk areas. While yellow fever is transmitted by mosquito bite, the use of mosquito nets is only recommended to avoid the transmission of mosquito-borne diseases for which there is no effective immunization. (NMS M&ID, 3rd Ed. p. 84, 299–302, 384).

32. The answer is E. If we consider that most viruses penetrate the organism by adsorption to mucosal surfaces or injection by a vector, it follows that any virus that causes a disease characterized by a disseminated skin rash must spread via the circulation. Papillomaviruses, rhinoviruses, and rotaviruses cause mucosal infections at the site of adsorption. HSV infects the sensory ganglia and, when the infection is reactivated, spreads centrifugally to the skin following the sensory nerves. (NMS M&ID, 3rd Ed. p. 241–4, 277–9)

33. The answer is D. Amantadine and rimantadine are two antiviral drugs that can be used prophylactically and therapeutically in influenza A infections. Both drugs bind to the M2 protein of the viral envelope, which appears to play a critical role in the uncoating step that precedes the release of the viral nucleic acid in the cytoplasm. In the presence of these drugs, uncoating does not take place. All other choices refer to steps of the influenza A virus replication cycle not affected by amantadine or rimantadine. (NMS M&ID, 3rd Ed. p. 211–2, 234)

34. The answer is C. The discovery that most rhinovirus strains use ICAM-1 as a receptor to invade nasal mucosal cells led to the development of a recombinant form of ICAM-1, which can be aerosolized into the nose and protects against rhinovirus infection. (NMS M&ID, 3rd Ed. p. 212, 234)

35. The answer is E. A common characteristic of the replication of all (+)RNA viruses, including retroviruses, is their synthesis of large polyproteins that are postsynthetically processed by viral proteases into the different structural and other proteins necessary for the assembly of progeny virions. Integration is unique to retroviruses; budding is an exclusive property of enveloped viruses; replication, in most cases, takes place in the cytoplasm (retroviruses being the exception); and most also do not pack polymerases because (+)RNA (with the exception of retroviral RNA) can be read by the cell ribosomes as mRNA. (NMS M&ID, 3rd Ed. p. 211–23)

36. The answer is D. Both polio vaccines contain the three types of poliovirus and both induce circulating antibodies of the three major isotypes (IgG, IgA, and IgM). Only the oral, attenuated vaccine induces mucosal immunity and, therefore, can prevent intestinal colonization. The propagation to close contacts may be seen as helpful, by contributing to the development of "herd" immunity, but also as potentially dangerous, if the close contact happens to be an immunocompromised individual who develops polio. The very small risk of causing the disease with the attenuated vaccine makes it less safe than the inactivated vaccine (assuming that it is effectively inactivated). (NMS M&ID, 3rd Ed. p. 84, 242, 295; IMI 4th Ed., 226–8)

37. The answer is C. The acute leukemia viruses that carry active oncogenes in their genome, and the insertion and expression of one such active oncogene in the cell's genome are associated with malignant transformation. In contrast, oncogenes of the leukemia group cause transformation by a variety of mechanisms which have to do with mutation and overexpression of a cellular proto-oncogene, usually after a long latency period. (NMS M&ID, 3rd Ed. p. 258–61)

38. The answer is C. Parainfluenza virus type 1 is the most common cause of croup in children. Other parainfluenza viruses, influenza A virus, and respiratory syncytial virus can also cause croup, with less frequency. (NMS M&ID, 3rd Ed. p. 309, 313; PAInfDis., 4th. Ed. p. 246–8)

39. The answer is C. One of the most widely used tests for the diagnosis of infectious mononucleosis is the monospot test, based on the fact that the EBV seems to induce the synthesis of antibodies that cross-react with horse erythrocytes. The test is not very specific and does not allow one to distinguish between acute or past infection, but its simplicity makes it very suitable for office use and the results are obtained almost immediately. (NMS M&ID, 3rd Ed. p. 281)

40. The answer is D. The mechanism responsible for malignant transformation in patients infected with HTLV-1 is believed to be the modification of a nuclear binding protein—NFkB—by the HTLV-1 *tax* gene product. The modification results in increased activity, which in turn causes overexpression of cytokine genes and cytokine receptor genes, leading to uncontrolled lymphocyte proliferation. (NMS M&ID, 3rd Ed. p. 259–60, IMI 4th Ed., 572–3)

41. The answer is B. The only titers that show a significant (fourfold) increase are those of antibodies against the varicella-zoster virus, which is the cause of chickenpox. Chickenpox is clinically associated with a vesicular rash, and can be particularly severe in immunocompromised children. (NMS M&ID, 3rd Ed. p. 273, 279–80, 493–4)

42. The answer is C. An attenuated vaccine to prevent chickenpox has been recently approved by the Food and Drug Administration (FDA) for routine administration to children, starting at 1 year of age. Note that most viral vaccines currently used are attenuated, followed in frequency by inactivated vaccines and recombinant proteins. Immune γ-globulin can be used to prevent the disease after exposure, but does not confer long-lasting protection. (NMS M&ID, 3rd Ed. p. 279–80, 493–4)

43. The answer is E. The question is basically asking which one of the listed viruses is a (−)RNA virus, because those viruses need to pack an RNA-dependent RNA polymerase in the virion to be able to replicate. DNA viruses (HBV, HSV) do not require this enzyme; neither do (+)RNA viruses (poliovirus). HIV packs a reverse transcriptase, which is an RNA-dependent DNA polymerase. (NMS M&ID, 3rd Ed. p. 211–23)

44. The answer is D. Progressive multifocal leukoencephalopathy (PML) is caused by the JC virus, a DNA virus of the papova group that is highly prevalent and appears to remain latent in most individuals. PML is virtually a disease of immunocompromised individuals, such as patients with acquired immune deficiency syndrome (AIDS), on which the latent virus starts to proliferate and infects glial cells that cause degeneration of the white matter. HIV could be described as a (+)RNA virus that has special affinity for microglial cells, but does not cause PML. Subacute sclerosing panencephalitis (SSPE) is caused by a defective form of measles virus that evades the immune system and causes persistent infection of neural cells. HSV can be described as an enveloped DNA virus that latently infects neural cells and is reactivated under stressful conditions. When it propagates to the CNS, it causes an acute encephalitis. Finally, kuru and Creutzfeldt-Jakob disease can be described as spongiform encephalopathy caused by an atypical agent. (NMS M&ID, 3rd Ed. p. 441–6)

45. The answer is D. Many viruses can affect the liver and cause jaundice. Among the (+)RNA viruses, the one most likely to cause jaundice in temperate climates is the hepatitis A virus (both the yellow fever virus and the hepatitis E virus are rarely involved as causes of jaundice in temperate climates). The mode of transmission of the hepatitis A and E viruses is fecal–oral; that is, the disease is acquired by ingesting contaminated food or water. The yellow fever virus is transmitted by mosquitoes. (NMS M&ID, 3rd Ed. p. 323–4, 331–2, 299–302, 482)

46. The answer is C. Transformed cells are immortalized; that is, they continue dividing indefinitely, and are in a state of metabolic activation. For that reason, they require an increased uptake of glucose. The expression of glycoproteins in the membrane is increased, and transformed cells are easier to agglutinate with lectins than normal cells. In contrast, the requirement for exogenous growth factors (such as those provided in serum) is lower. The expression of MHC molecules is usually decreased. (NMS M&ID, 3rd Ed. p. 251–2)

47. The answer is E. Several HSV mutations can account for resistance to acyclovir and related drugs, but the most common is thymidine kinase deficiency. Strains lacking the enzyme do not phosphorylate acyclovir, which remains inactive. Those strains are usually of reduced pathogenicity but can cause severe infections in immunocompromised patients. Mutation of the viral DNA polymerase, reducing its affinity for fully phosphorylated acyclovir, is another HSV resistance mechanism, considerably less frequent than lack of thymidine kinase. (NMS M&ID, 3rd Ed. p. 239)

48. The answer is B. Type I interferons inhibit viral protein synthesis by two mechanisms: induction of an adenine nucleotide with RNAse activity and inactivation of the elongation/initiation factor-2 (NMS M&ID, 3rd Ed. p. 233). All other choices could inhibit viral replication, but type I interferons are not known to cause any of these abnormalities.

49. The answer is E. Plaque formation involves cell lysis, and that is a consequence of viral replication, particularly in the case of naked viruses that need to lyse the host cell for the progeny to be released. This is only possible if an active viral infection has taken place in the cell monolayer. Hemadsorption detects infected cells expressing viral hemagglutinins on the membrane, but fails to give information concerning the release of infectious particles from those cells. The remaining assays detect viral antigens or viral sequences, but also fail to indicate whether infectious particles are being released. (NMS M&ID, 3rd Ed. p. 271–3)

50. The answer is A. The organ damage seen in chronic viral hepatitis is believed to result from the immune response directed against persistently infected hepatocytes. The viral infection by itself seems to be of limited cytopathogenicity, and immune-mediated damage seems to be primarily responsible for tissue damage. In contrast, the viral cytopathic effect is primarily responsible for the extensive liver damage in fulminant viral hepatitis. In the other conditions listed, there may be contributions both from viral cytopathogenicity and inflammation secondary to the immune response against viral infected cells in causing cell and tissue damage, but in those cases the role of the immune response is not as significant as in the case of chronic viral hepatitis, with the possible exception of leukocytic choriomeningitis, a rare form of viral meningitis caused by an arenavirus. (NMS M&ID, 3rd Ed. p. 319, 266, 486).

51. The answer is A. Although most viral diseases with vesicular rash are caused by dsDNA viruses of the herpes group, the clinical picture described in the vignette suggests herpangina, caused by type A coxsackieviruses, which are (+)RNA enteroviruses. The enanthem associated with measles—caused by a (−)RNA paramyxovirus—is classically described as a tiny, punctuate, whitish rash with erythematous base localized to the buccal mucosa, above the lower molars. Herpesviruses and parvoviruses can cause febrile diseases in children, but parvovirus infections are not associated with vesicular rash, and the vesicular rashes associated with viruses of the herpes groups tend to be disseminated and affect the skin, rather than the mucosae. (NMS M&ID, 3rd Ed. p. 277–80, 290–2, 296, 311).

52. The answer is D. While some of the early gene products of adenovirus block the expression of MHC-I molecules, all of these viruses share the property of coding for proteins—polyoma T antigen, the E6 transforming gene of papilloma virus, and the E1B protein of adenovirus—which inactivate p53, thus disabling one of the major cellular mechanisms of protection against mutation. The polyoma virus middle T antigen and some retroviral antigens (e.g., *v-erb*) activate membrane-associated protein kinases. EBNA-5 and EBNA-2 form a complex that activates a G1 cyclin and *c-myc* promotes cell entry into cycle (NMS M&ID, 3rd Ed. p. 252–5).

53. The answer is E. Both vaccines are equally efficient in inducing systemic antibodies of all isotypes (including IgG neutralizing antibodies and IgA antibodies), and both prevent viremic spread to the nervous system. Only the oral vaccine, prepared with attenuated virus, will result in the fecal excretion of live virus, which can be spread to nonimmunized close contacts by the fecal-oral route. None of the vaccines will elicit hemagglutination-inhibiting antibodies because picornaviruses do not have viral hemagglutinins, found mostly in orthomyxoviruses and paramyxoviruses. (NMS M&ID, 3rd Ed. p. 295, 305–6, 309; IMI 4th Ed., p. 227).

54. The answer is B. While most Hantaviruses cause hemorrhagic fevers and acute kidney failure, the Sin Nombre (*Four Corners*) strain causes acute respiratory failure with high mortality. Hemorrhagic fever, meningitis, and influenza-like syndromes can be caused by a variety of other viruses, including members of the arenavirus family. (NMS M&ID, 3rd Ed. p. 319–20).

55. The answer is A. The replication cycle of HSV (as that of most DNA viruses) is initiated by cellular DNA-dependent RNA polymerases that read about a third of the viral genome and transcribe mRNA segments coding for the early proteins, which include a viral DNA-dependent DNA polymerase and other regulatory proteins. This sequence of events precedes genomic replication; hence, in the given scenario it would happen in the first 6 hours of infection. The capsid proteins and all other late proteins are transcribed by modified cell polymerases using progeny DNA as template. Acyclovir has no effect on the initial transcription of early genes, but this drug blocks DNA synthesis. Therefore, late genes will not be expressed and capsid proteins will not be synthesized. (NMS M&ID, 3rd Ed. p. 212–18).

56. The answer is A. Some diagnoses require knowledge of both clinical symptoms and epidemiology to be considered. Given the acute onset of presentation of this disease in an individual traveling from South America, consideration of diseases prevalent in the Southern hemisphere appears in order. Although viral influenza knows no borders, the degree and intensity of the pain and the presence of a maculopapular rash suggest that this is not a simple case of flu. On the other hand, a dengue epidemic has been raging in the northern part of South America. Being a mosquito-borne disease, dengue is more prevalent in areas of low altitude and high humidity, such as Cartagena, situated in the Caribbean coast of Colombia. The clinical symptoms include all those referred by the patient. Because bleeding is not part of this patient's symptoms, yellow fever and Machupo hemorrhagic fever (more common in Bolivia than in Colombia) are not as likely diagnoses. (NMS M&ID, 3rd Ed. p. 299–302; 319–20).

57. The answer is D. The replication of DNA viruses is blocked if DNA synthesis is blocked. Although viral DNA can be partially transcribed by the cell DNA-dependent RNA polymerases and early proteins are then translated from those early mRNAs, the transcription and translation of full genomes are achieved only after progeny DNA synthesis is synthesized. In other words, late proteins (which include most structural proteins needed to build progeny virus) are not synthesized if the synthesis of progeny DNA is inhibited. Of all the viruses listed, only herpes viruses have a DNA genome. (NMS M&ID, 3rd Ed. p. 209, 211–4)

58. The answer is A. Ara-A, one of the earliest antiviral agents described, is a nucleoside analog that is incorporated into a nascent DNA chain but lacks the hydroxyl group that is required for cross-linking to the next nucleoside; therefore the DNA chain is terminated. This results in inhibition of progeny DNA synthesis and, consequently, on the inability to synthesize late proteins, including capsid proteins. All other proteins listed as choices are early proteins, synthesized from the original DNA of the infecting virus. (NMS M&ID, 3rd Ed. p. 217–8, 236–7, 254)

59. The answer is A. The question could be rephrased as "which one of the following viruses is a DNA virus?" because DNA synthesis is essential for DNA virus replication, but is not essential for the replication of most RNA viruses. EBV, also known as human herpesvirus 4, is the only DNA virus on the list. (NMS M&ID, 3rd Ed. p. 209, 211–14)

60. The answer is D. All the listed diseases are caused by DNA viruses, and the viruses that cause four of them belong to the human herpesvirus (HHV) group: chickenpox (varicella-zoster virus, HHV 3), infectious mononucleosis (CMV, HHV 4), Kaposi's sarcoma (HHV 8), and roseola infantum or exanthema subitum (HHV 6). In contrast, molluscum contagiosum is caused by an unclassified poxvirus. (NMS M&ID, 3rd Ed. p. 277–83, 291, 523)

Mycology and Parasitology

Test 4

Mycology and Parasitology

LIST OF COMMON ABBREVIATIONS

AIDS   acquired immunodeficiency syndrome
ATP   adenosine 5′-triphosphate
CBC   complete blood count
CSF   cerebrospinal fluid

DNA   deoxyribonucleic acid
HIV   human immunodeficiency virus
KOH   potassium hydroxide

Directions: (Items 1–50) Each of the numbered items or incomplete statements in this section is followed by answers or by completions of the statement. Select the ONE lettered answer or completion that is BEST in each case.

QUESTIONS 1–2

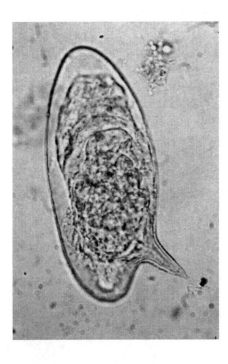

A Spanish-speaking migrant worker is seen with complaints of chronic, intermittent bloody diarrhea for about 1 year. On physical examination hepatosplenomegaly is detected. A peripheral blood examination shows eosinophilia. His serum transaminases are elevated. An upper gastrointestinal series reveals esophageal varices. Bacteriologic study of the feces shows normal flora. A search for eggs and parasites in the feces reveals the organism shown in the figure.

1. The acquisition of this disease involves

   (A) Bite by *Anopheles* mosquitoes
   (B) Deposition of fecal material containing infective forms on the bite site of triatomine bugs
   (C) Ingestion of contaminated pork meat
   (D) Ingestion of watercress grown in areas irrigated by water contaminated with infective cercaria
   (E) Larval penetration through the skin while swimming or wading in infested waters

2. The drug of choice to treat this infection is one that

   (A) Inactivates the antioxidant defenses of the parasite
   (B) Blocks glucose transport into the parasite
   (C) Interferes with parasite locomotion
   (D) Uncouples oxidative phosphorylation and interrupts glycolysis
   (E) Interferes with mitochondrial oxidation

QUESTIONS 3–5

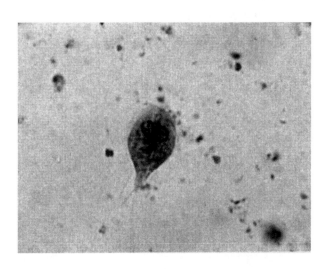

A 19-year-old white woman temporarily employed at a day care center has suffered for the last 5 days with an increasingly debilitating diarrhea with cramps and borborygmi. Her stools are frequent, often explosive, fermentative, and foul smelling. Past history reveals that the patient enjoys hiking in the mountains and that she had camped around Vail, CO, 2 weeks before the onset of her diarrhea. A physical examination reveals a distressed but otherwise apparently fit young woman. Temperature is 99.1°F, pulse 78/minute, blood pressure 115/65 mm Hg, with slightly increased respiration rate. Ocular, oral, and chest examinations are all normal. There is mild abdominal tenderness but no enlargement of liver or spleen. Trichrome stain of the sediment of a fecal extract reveals the organism reproduced in the figure.

3. Which is the main pathogenic mechanism responsible for this patient's diarrhea?

   (A) Interference with the absorptive functions of duodenal villi

   (B) Invasion and toxic damage of the mucosa

   (C) Invasion of the draining lymphatics, causing backflow into the intestine

   (D) Secretion of proteases that destroy the intestinal villi

   (E) Stimulation of electrolyte secretion by mucosal cells in the small intestine

4. To treat this patient's diarrhea, the most indicated therapy would be

   (A) Administration of oral metronidazole

   (B) Administration of oral trimethoprim-sulfamethoxazole

   (C) Administration of oral iodoquinol

   (D) Symptomatic measures only (bland diet and sports drink)

   (E) Intravenous fluid and electrolyte replacement

5. Which of the following characteristics of the infectious agent causing this patient's diarrhea has a more significant impact on the choice of an effective antimicrobial to treat her?

   (A) Anaerobic metabolism

   (B) Fecal-oral transmission

   (C) Motility

   (D) Resistance to acid pH

   (E) Resistance to low concentrations of chlorine

6. A 5-year-old boy is seen in a family care office because of a rectal prolapse. The mother claims that the child has been healthy since birth, but 2 weeks before started complaining of diarrhea alternating with tenesmus, which got progressively worse and did not respond to dietary changes. Several white worms, about 3–5 cm long, which appear to have one extremity burrowing into the rectal mucosa, are seen by visual inspection. This child is likely to be infected with

   (A) *Ancylostoma duodenale*

   (B) *Ascaris lumbricoides*

   (C) *Enterobius vermicularis*

   (D) *Trichinella spiralis*

   (E) *Trichuris trichiura*

7. A 7-year-old boy from Sumter, SC, is taken to the emergency room in September. The family gives the history of sudden disease starting 24 hours earlier when the boy felt dizzy and disoriented, with a strong headache. He went to bed and fell into a deep sleep from which he could not be awakened in the morning. He had been well and active, having participated in an outing to the nearby lakes the Sunday before he felt sick. A patient with this presentation is likely infected with

   (A) *Balantidium coli*

   (B) *Entamoeba histolytica*

   (C) *Giardia lamblia*

   (D) *Naegleria fowleri*

   (E) *Toxoplasma gondii*

QUESTIONS 8–9

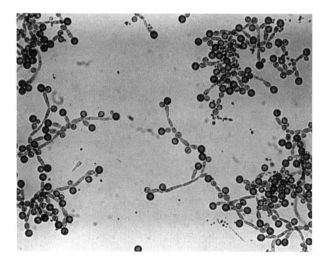

A 56-year-old man receiving chemotherapy for metastatic prostate carcinoma develops persistent fever not affected by administration of broad-spectrum antibiotics. A CBC and differential reveals profound neutropenia and a white exudate is seen in the vitreous of the right eye. The organism shown in the figure was grown from the peripheral blood in Sabouraud's agar.

8. This patient's blood has been invaded by

(A) *Aspergillus fumigatus*
(B) *Candida albicans*
(C) *Coccidioides immitis*
(D) *Cryptosporidium*
(E) *Malassezia furfur*

9. The drug of choice to treat this patient would be one that

(A) Binds to ergosterol and disrupts the cell membrane
(B) Blocks squalene epoxidase
(C) Blocks the synthesis of fecosterol
(D) Inhibits cell division
(E) Interferes with the synthesis of 14-dimethyl-lanosterol

10. Which of the following developmental stages of *Ascaris lumbricoides* is responsible for the development of Loeffler's syndrome in infected patients?

(A) Cyst formation in intercostal muscles
(B) Extra-intestinal migration involving temporary residence in the lung
(C) Hematogenous dissemination from the skin to the lungs
(D) Penetration of the intestinal wall and migration to the liver
(E) Retrograde migration from the intestine to the stomach, esophagus, throat, and lungs

11. The most reliable evidence for the diagnosis of an active systemic fungal infection is given by

(A) A characteristic pattern of chest radiograph
(B) A positive complement-fixation test
(C) A positive skin test
(D) Culture and identification of the fungus from adequate specimens
(E) Identification of a source of potential exposure

12. In a case of suspected tinea versicolor, the diagnosis is easily confirmed by

(A) Detecting precipitating antibodies by double immunodiffusion
(B) Exposure to ultraviolet light
(C) Response to topical application of tolnaftate
(D) Culture in Sabouraud's agar
(E) Direct microscopy of KOH preparations of affected skin scrapings

QUESTIONS 13–14

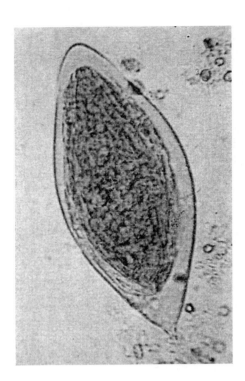

An Ethiopian taxi driver in Washington, DC, complains of intermittent hematuria and progressive difficulties in passing urine. The organism reproduced in the figure is visualized on his urinary sediment.

13. This patient acquired his infection by

(A) Eating contaminated pork
(B) Sexual intercourse
(C) Bathing in infested waters
(D) Drinking contaminated water
(E) Eating improperly prepared sushi

14. This patient is at risk of developing

(A) Anemia
(B) Bladder carcinoma
(C) Esophageal varices
(D) Kidney insufficiency
(E) Urethral stenosis

QUESTIONS 15–16

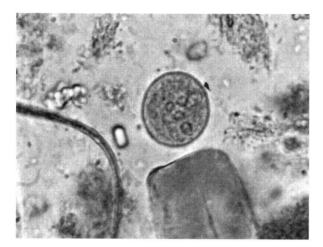

A 22-year-old man from Brazil who has been living in New York for the last year has developed chronic diarrhea (sometimes bloody), fever, hepatomegaly, and weight loss. The following organism (in the figure) was visualized on an ova and parasite (O&P) examination of the feces with an iodine stain.

15. This organism is most likely

(A) *Balantidium coli*
(B) *Entamoeba coli*
(C) *Entamoeba hartmanni*
(D) *Entamoeba histolytica*
(E) *Giardia lamblia*

16. The drug of choice to treat this patient is

(A) Amphotericin B
(B) Doxycycline
(C) Iodoquinol
(D) Metronidazole
(E) Quinacrine hydrochloride

QUESTIONS 17–18

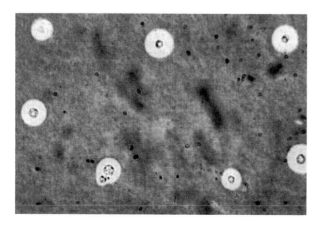

A 21-year-old Hispanic woman with systemic lupus erythematosus presents with symptoms of meningitis. The CSF protein is elevated and the glucose is low. The Gram stain shows no organisms. The result of an India ink preparation is shown in the figure.

17. This organism can be recovered in large quantities from

(A) Bat guano
(B) Blackbird roosting grounds
(C) Mexican pottery
(D) Organic debris
(E) Pigeon and chicken droppings

18. The main virulence factor of this organism is its

(A) Ability to survive intracellularly
(B) Antiphagocytic capsule
(C) Cell wall lipopolysaccharide
(D) Poor immunogenicity
(E) Resistance to most antimicrobials

QUESTIONS 19–21

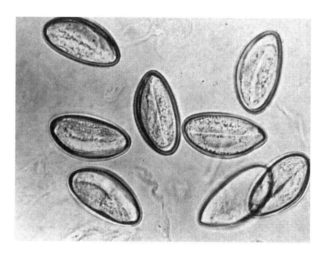

A 3-year-old boy complains of intense pruritus ani, particularly at bedtime. The organism shown in the figure is recovered from a scotch tape applied to the perianal region.

19. In deciding how to treat this infection, it is most important to remember that

(A) Females lay eggs in the perianal region at night
(B) It requires an intermediate host for transmission to humans
(C) It is highly contagious because the eggs are easily disseminated
(D) Main symptoms are caused by intestinal irritation or obstruction
(E) The eggs are embryonated

20. Which of the following drugs is indicated for the treatment of this infection?

(A) Bithionol
(B) Ivermectin
(C) Mebendazole
(D) Niclosamide
(E) Thiabendazole

21. The antimicrobial drug you would prescribe for the patient is one that

(A) Disrupts microtubule formation and glucose transport
(B) Disrupts microtubules and inhibits fumarate reductase
(C) Inhibits glutathione-S-transferase
(D) Interrupts neuromuscular activity
(E) Uncouples oxidative phosphorylation

QUESTIONS 22–24

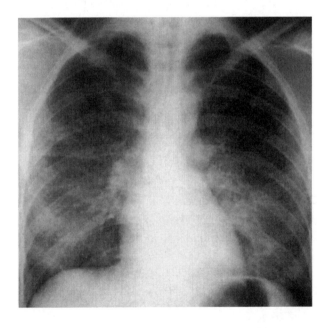

A 32-year-old white man is seen at the emergency room with shortness of breath and cyanosis. The chest radiograph is shown in the figure. A bronchoalveolar lavage sediment stained by methenamine-silver reveals cysts with multiple spores. The patient is found to be HIV-positive.

22. Treatment of this patient's pulmonary infection should involve administering an antimicrobial drug or combination of drugs that

(A) Blocks mRNA translation
(B) Blocks the 50S ribosome
(C) Inhibits HIV replication
(D) Interferes with nucleotide synthesis
(E) Prevents peptidoglycan cross-linking

23. Treatment of this patient's HIV infection may be delayed until his pneumonia is controlled because

(A) Antiretrovirals interfere with the activity of the drugs used to treat the pneumonia
(B) Both zidovudine (AZT) and the drugs used to treat the pneumonia are hepatotoxic
(C) The drugs used to treat the pneumonia affect the pharmacokinetics of antiretroviral agents
(D) The pharmacokinetics of the drugs used to treat the pneumonia are affected by antiretroviral agents
(E) AZT and the drugs used to treat the pneumonia can have a synergistic effect, causing bone marrow depression

24. Disseminated cryptococcal infection is MOST common in

(A) AIDS
(B) Bone marrow aplasia
(C) Chronic granulomatous disease
(D) Infantile agammaglobulinemia
(E) Neutropenia

25. The prevention of recurrences of cryptococcal meningitis in patients with AIDS involves administering an antimycotic agent that

(A) Blocks mRNA translation
(B) Disrupts cell membranes
(C) Inhibits ergosterol incorporation in cell membranes
(D) Inhibits ergosterol synthesis
(E) Interferes with microtubule assembly during cell division

26. Which one of the following fungi is isolated more frequently from human samples in the clinical laboratories of industrialized countries?

(A) *Candida albicans*
(B) *Cryptococcus neoformans*
(C) *Histoplasma capsulatum*
(D) *Sporothrix schenckii*
(E) *Trichophyton rubrum*

27. *Plasmodia* responsible for a specific case of malaria generally are identified by

  (A) Cultural characteristics of the organisms on media containing red blood cells
  (B) Morphological characteristics of the organisms in samples of infected blood
  (C) The latent period of the exoerythrocytic cycle
  (D) The protozoa immobilization test (PIT) with specific antisera
  (E) The results of an hepatic biopsy searching for hypnozoites

28. What causes the characteristic relapses of African trypanosomiasis?

  (A) Antigenic mimicry of host material by the trypanosome
  (B) Poor immunogenicity of the parasite
  (C) Inadequate therapy
  (D) Periodic release of trypanosomes from red blood cells
  (E) Sequential antigenic variation of the trypanosome surface glycoprotein

29. Most antimycotic drugs target fungal

  (A) Cell membrane integrity
  (B) DNA polymerases
  (C) Enzymes involved in ergosterol synthesis
  (D) Microtubules
  (E) Ribosomes

30. A 45-year-old male missionary was flown from Honduras to the United States with a severe crisis of malaria. His relevant history included a mild anemia secondary to glucose-6-phosphate dehydrogenase deficiency, and malaria diagnosed 4 months earlier and treated with chloroquine, which relapsed last week. After admission he is started on a combination of chloroquine and primaquine. Twenty-four hours later the patient's condition worsened, his temperature rose to 41°C, his urine became very dark, and his urinary output declined to about 50 mL/day (normal: 1500 mL/day). The deterioration of this patient's condition was most likely caused by

  (A) Acute dehydration
  (B) Acute hemolysis caused by primaquine toxicity
  (C) Bilirubin toxicity
  (D) Deposition of immune complexes in the glomeruli
  (E) Massive release of merozoites from infected red cells

31. The cause of anemia associated with ancylostomiasis is

  (A) Bone marrow depression caused by parasitic invasion
  (B) Lack of vitamin B_{12} from competition in its absorption by the parasite
  (C) Malabsorption of folic acid because of chronic diarrhea
  (D) Massive hemoptysis during the early stages of parasitic maturation
  (E) Persistent iron loss

32. Which of the following fungi is most likely to spread from person to person?

  (A) *Aspergillus fumigatus*
  (B) *Cryptococcus neoformans*
  (C) *Epidermophyton floccosum*
  (D) *Histoplasma capsulatum*
  (E) *Sporothrix schenckii*

33. Which one of the following clinical and laboratory findings is highly unusual in Chagas' disease?

  (A) An erythematous nodule at the site of an insect bite
  (B) Numerous C-shaped organisms in the peripheral blood during the late phase of the disease
  (C) Fever, chills, anorexia
  (D) Unilateral swelling of upper eyelid and contiguous areas (Romaña's sign)
  (E) Hepatosplenomegaly and late cardiac involvement

34. *Plasmodium vivax* has which unique epidemiological and laboratory characteristic?

  (A) Duffy-negative individuals are resistant to infection
  (B) Gametocytes can be seen in the peripheral blood
  (C) Persistent infection of hepatic cells by hypnozoites
  (D) Ring forms can be seen in infected red blood cells
  (E) Transmission via contaminated blood or needle

35. A 48-year-old Mexican farm worker from Arizona presents with a history of cough, intermittent fever, and hemoptysis, which has persisted for several months and has been associated with weight loss. His condition has recently worsened, with complaints of persistent severe headaches in addition to the remaining symptoms. Which of the following fungi is most likely responsible for this patient's disease?

(A) *Blastomyces dermatitidis*
(B) *Candida tropicalis*
(C) *Coccidioides immitis*
(D) *Cryptococcus neoformans*
(E) *Histoplasma capsulatum*

36. If an elderly African-American farmer from the Southeast United States has chronic productive cough and slowly progressive skin ulcers, suspect a fungal infection with

(A) *Blastomyces dermatitidis*
(B) *Coccidioides immitis*
(C) *Cryptococcus neoformans*
(D) *Histoplasma capsulatum*
(E) *Sporothrix schenckii*

37. Which of the following clinical or laboratory features is frequently found in patients with **mild** forms of visceral larva migrans?

(A) Endophthalmitis
(B) Eosinophilia
(C) Portal hypertension
(D) Pulmonary infiltrates
(E) Splenomegaly

38. The main source of human infection with *Blastomyces dermatitidis* is

(A) Arthrospores carried by strong winds
(B) Domestic animals
(C) Dried bird fecal material
(D) Human carriers
(E) Organic debris

39. To confirm a diagnosis of tinea unguium, you would prefer to

(A) Culture nail scrapings in Sabouraud's agar followed by speciation by morphological characteristics
(B) Evaluate the systemic administration of itraconazole
(C) Expose the affected nail to Wood's light in a darkened room
(D) Look for anti-*Trichophyton* antibodies in peripheral blood
(E) Perform direct microscopy of KOH preparations of affected nail scrapings

40. A 47-year-old woman presents with a cutaneous lesion 2 cm in diameter. The surface is verrucous and has been present for 3 years. A biopsy shows a thickening of the stratum corneum, many giant cells, and brown sclerotic bodies. The most effective treatment for this disease is

(A) Amphotericin B
(B) Fluconazole
(C) Itraconazole
(D) Surgical excision
(E) Oral potassium iodide

41. The most dependable evidence for the diagnosis of an active systemic fungal infection comes from

(A) Culture and/or identification of the fungus from adequate specimens
(B) India ink test on CSF
(C) KOH preparation of skin scrapings
(D) Serological assay of circulating antibodies
(E) Skin tests with fungal extracts

42. In the United States, toxoplasmosis is most commonly transmitted by

(A) Close contact with an asymptomatic carrier
(B) Ingestion of food contaminated by rodent excreta
(C) Ingestion of merozoites in undercooked meat from infected animals
(D) Ingestion of oocysts excreted by infected cats
(E) Inhalation of aerosolized eggs

43. The most common source of infection for *Anisakis marina* is

(A) Crustaceans
(B) Free-living larvae
(C) Lightly seared frozen squid
(D) Lightly smoked salmon
(E) Oysters

44. In humans, which of the following stages is characteristic of the life cycle of *Ascaris lumbricoides?*

(A) Cyst formation in striated muscle
(B) Extra-intestinal migration involving temporary residence in the lung
(C) Penetration of the intestinal wall and migration to the liver across the peritoneal cavity
(D) Retrograde migration from the intestine to the stomach, esophagus, throat, and lungs
(E) Sexual reproduction inside the intestine and larval dissemination through the bloodstream

45. *Trichomonas vaginalis* is most commonly transmitted by

- (A) Contact with surfaces containing cysts resistant to dryness
- (B) Fecal–oral transfer of trophozoites from an infected carrier
- (C) Cysts acquired from an infected partner during intercourse
- (D) Trophozoites acquired from an infected partner during intercourse
- (E) Viable trophozoites acquired through the use of moist towels and bathroom utensils

46. *Malassezia furfur* tends to cause systemic infections in infants receiving parenteral nutrition because

- (A) Indwelling catheters are easily colonized by skin pathogens
- (B) *M. furfur* is a common skin pathogen
- (C) Parenteral fluids are often contaminated with skin pathogens
- (D) The immune system of those infants is deficient
- (E) This organism requires long-chain fatty acids for growth

QUESTIONS 47–48

A 48-year-old white man seeks medical care because of generalized muscle pains and periorbital edema. Physical examination shows that the large muscular masses are tender to palpation and splinter hemorrhages are noted on the nail beds of several fingers. The patient is an avid sportsman and he recently traveled to Maine for bear hunting. He is also an avid fisherman, and after his trip to Maine he visited the Bahamas, where he caught sailfish and swordfish.

47. Which of the following diagnoses appears most likely in this patient?

- (A) Trichinellosis
- (B) Anisakiasis
- (C) Strongyloidiasis
- (D) Trichuriasis
- (E) Diphyllobothriasis

48. Which of the following diagnostic procedures would most likely confirm the clinical diagnosis?

- (A) CBC and differential
- (B) Examination of the stool for ova
- (C) Gram stain of feces
- (D) Muscle biopsy
- (E) Serological assay of anti-*Trichinella* antibodies

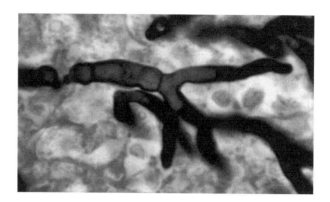

49. A 65-year-old male veteran seeks medical attention because of persistent dry cough for the previous 4 weeks. He had been feeling relatively well, and denies fever and weight loss. His personal antecedents include pulmonary tuberculosis at age 20, and he has smoked about 1 pack of cigarettes a day since he was 18. After radiograph of the chest was taken, the patient was operated on to remove a nodular mass from the lower left lobe. The figure reproduces a section of that mass stained with methenamine-silver. The organism infecting this patient is

- (A) *Aspergillus*
- (B) *Malassezia furfur*
- (C) *Mucor*
- (D) *Nocardia*
- (E) *Rhizopus*

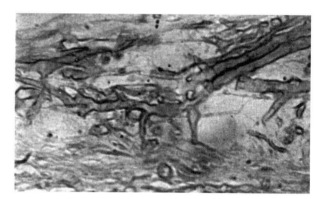

50. A 37-year-old diabetic woman from Ecuador is admitted to a tertiary hospital in a ketoacidotic state. Her serum glucose level is 325 mg/dL. Physical examination shows moderate exophthalmos. A white, cottony growth is seen in the nares. A KOH preparation of this material is shown in the figure. This patient has

- (A) Actinomycosis
- (B) Aspergillosis
- (C) Blastomycosis
- (D) Paracoccidioidomycosis
- (E) Zygomycosis (mucormycosis)

TEST 4: Mycology and Parasitology

1. E	11. D	21. A	31. E	41. A
2. A	12. E	22. D	32. C	42. D
3. A	13. C	23. E	33. B	43. D
4. A	14. B	24. A	34. A	44. B
5. A	15. D	25. D	35. C	45. D
6. E	16. D	26. A	36. A	46. E
7. D	17. E	27. B	37. B	47. A
8. B	18. B	28. E	38. E	48. D
9. A	19. C	29. C	39. E	49. A
10. B	20. C	30. B	40. C	50. E

ANSWERS AND EXPLANATIONS

Note: Page numbers designated as "IMI 4th Ed" refer to *Introduction to Medical Immunology,* 4th ed., New York/Basel, Marcel Dekker, 1998. Page numbers designated as "NMS M&ID 3rd Ed" refer to *NMS Microbiology and Infectious Diseases,* 3rd ed. Baltimore, Williams & Wilkins, 1997. Page numbers indicated as "PAInfDis 4th Ed" refer to Reese RE, Betts RF, eds., *Practical Approach to Infectious Diseases,* 4th ed., Boston, Little, Brown & Co., 1996.

1. The answer is E. The clinical picture suggests an infection that may involve both the gastrointestinal tract and the liver. The finding of an oval egg with a lateral spike is diagnostic of *Schistosoma mansoni,* an organism that infects both the liver and the mesenteric vessels, causing hepatic disease, portal hypertension, and chronic bloody diarrhea from the passage of eggs through the intestinal wall into the feces. The infection is acquired by swimming or wading in water containing free-swimming cercariae that burrow through the skin and penetrate the circulation, spreading initially to the liver and from there migrate back to the mesenteric vessels. The other modes of infection correspond to different parasites: Plasmodia are transmitted by mosquito bites, triatomine bugs carry *Trypanosoma cruzi,* ingestion of contaminated pork meat can result in acquisition of *Taenia solium* and *Trichinella spiralis,* ingestion of contaminated watercress is the usual way to acquire *Fasciola hepatica.* (NMS M&ID, 3rd Ed. p. 402–4)

2. The answer is A. The drug of choice for treating schistosomiasis is praziquantel, which inactivates the parasite's antioxidant enzyme glutathione-S-oxidase. Mebendazole, used for the treatment of many nematode infections, blocks glucose transport into the parasite. Pyrantel, used to treat nematode infections, causes neuromuscular paralysis in the parasite and is one of several antinematode agents that interfere with the parasite's locomotion. Niclosamide, used for treating cestode infections, uncouples oxidative phosphorylation and electron transport reactions at the mitochondrial level and inhibits ATP production. (NMS M&ID, 3rd Ed. p. 368–9, 404)

3. The answer is A. The clinical picture, the travel history to one of the known endemic areas for *Giardia lamblia* in the United States (another well known endemic area is St. Petersburg in Russia), and the result of the examination of fecal material establish a diagnosis of giardiasis. *G. lamblia* is not invasive and not known to release toxins; it is believed to cause diarrhea by interfering with the absorptive functions of duodenal villi by a mechanism that is not fully understood. (NMS M&ID, 3rd Ed. p. 374–6)

4. The answer is A. Metronidazole (Flagyl) is the drug of choice for the treatment of giardiasis. Quinacrine hydrochloride is also effective, but iodoquinol is usually used when treating amebiasis. Symptomatic measures are not sufficient and intravenous fluid replacement is usually unnecessary. (NMS M&ID, 3rd Ed. p. 365, 375–6)

5. The answer is A. Metronidazole is only effective after reduction, and this only happens in anaerobic organisms. Therefore, because *Giardia* is anaerobic, it is susceptible to metronidazole, which is one of the main reasons this is the drug of choice for this organism. (NMS M&ID, 3rd Ed. p. 48, 365).

6. The answer is E. The clinical symptoms, morphological characteristics, and habitat are suggestive of an infection with *Trichuris trichiura. Trichinella spiralis* encysts in muscles, and does not infect the intestine. *Enterobius vermicularis* is a smaller worm (1–3 mm) and the most typical symptom in infected patients is pruritus ani. *Ascaris lumbricoides* is a considerably larger worm (20–30 cm) and does not attach to the mucosa. *Ancylostoma duodenale* does not infect beyond the cecum and does not cause the described symptoms. (NMS M&ID, 3rd Ed. p. 389–94).

7. The answer is D. The clinical picture is suggestive of meningoencephalitis, and the possibility of infection with a freshwater-living organism should be considered. *Balantidium* and *Giardia* can be excluded because the infection associated with these parasites is localized to the gastrointestinal tract. *Entamoeba histolytica* may cause brain abscesses, but usually as a complication of chronic infection. *Toxoplasma* is not a water-living organism and is only associated with cerebral infections in chronically infected patients, disseminating from the large intestine to the liver, lungs, brain, and other locations. *Naegleria* is a free-living ameba, found in lakes and irrigation ditches in the southern states during the warm months and can infect the brain by penetrating through the cribriform plate. (NMS M&ID, 3rd Ed. p. 371–82).

8. The answer is B. The scenario of a patient receiving chemotherapy and developing neutropenia and fever that does not respond to antibiotics should be familiar as suggesting systemic candidiasis. The white exudate seen in the vitreous of the right eye could correspond to endophthalmitis caused by *Candida*. The morphologic characteristic seen in the organism isolated from the blood (round yeasts with germ tubes) is also characteristic of *Candida*. (NMS M&ID, 3rd Ed. p. 347–8; PAInfDis, 4th Ed. p. 663–4)

9. The answer is A. Treatment of systemic candidiasis usually requires administration of amphotericin B, while treatment of mucosal candidiasis can be done with a variety of drugs, including nystatin and the azoles. The mechanism of action of nystatin and amphotericin is basically identical, but nystatin is not absorbed when given orally and cannot be administered intravenously, so it is not suitable for treatment of systemic infections. The listed mechanisms of action correspond to allylamines (block squalene epoxidase), morpholines (block the synthesis of fecosterol and episterol), griseofulvin (inhibit cell division), and azoles (interfere with the synthesis of 14-dimethyllanosterol). (NMS M&ID, 3rd Ed. p. 340–2).

10. The answer is B. *Ascaris* infection is acquired by ingestion of eggs, which hatch in the intestine. The larvae burrow through the intestinal wall, enter the blood or lymphatic circulation, and reach the lungs, where they molt twice. From the lung parenchyma they migrate to the trachea and esophagus, and eventually reach the intestine, where they reproduce and lay eggs. Formation of cysts in striated muscle is characteristic of *Trichinella spiralis,* hematogenous dissemination from the skin is typical of *Necator* and *Ancylostoma*, migration to the liver is typical of *Schistosoma mansoni,* and retrograde migration from the stomach to the lungs is not seen with human parasites. (NMS M&ID, 3rd Ed. p. 390–4; 402–4).

11. The answer is D. The gold standard for diagnosis of fungal infections (and any other infections) is the culture and identification of the fungus from reliable specimens. Skin tests and complement-fixation tests give information that may be useful, but not as unquestionable (either type of test may be positive because of previous exposure, rather than reflect active infection). Radiograph patterns and identifying potential sources of infection are useful to suspect a diagnosis, but clearly insufficient to confirm it. (NMS M&ID, 3rd Ed. p. 339–40).

12. The answer is E. In the case of cutaneous mycoses, clinical features plus visualization of fungal structures in a KOH preparation is usually considered sufficient to establish a diagnosis, because the treatment does not depend so much on the precise identification of the fungal species involved. Tinea versicolor is easy to suspect because of the discoloration of the infected areas, and a KOH preparation of skin scrapings shows intertwined mycelia and budding yeasts (described as "spaghetti and meatballs"), which are characteristic of the etiologic agent, *Malassezia furfur*. (NMS M&ID, 3rd Ed. p. 339–40, 344).

13. The answer is C. The clinical picture of hematuria and difficulty in passing urine in an African patient is strongly suggestive of schistosomiasis; the diagnosis is confirmed by the finding of *Schistosoma haematobium* eggs in the urine. The infection is acquired by bathing or swimming in infested rivers or lakes. (NMS M&ID, 3rd Ed. p. 402–3)

14. The answer is B. *Schistosoma haematobium* infects the perivesical venous plexus and the parasite eggs burrow through the bladder and are eventually passed in the urine. The process of chronic inflammation of the bladder seems to create predisposing conditions for the development of bladder carcinoma. (NMS M&ID, 3rd Ed. p. 402–3)

15. The answer is D. The clinical picture—chronic diarrhea (sometimes bloody), fever, hepatomegaly, and weight loss—is suggestive of an organism that infects the colon (bloody diarrhea) and has disseminated to the liver (hepatomegaly) and probably has triggered an intense inflammatory reaction (fever and weight loss) compatible with amebiasis (intestinal and extraintestinal). The fecal examination reveals tetranucleated cyst, characteristic of *Entamoeba histolytica*. *Entamoeba coli* has cysts with eight nuclei and is a commensal. *Balantidium coli* is a ciliate and *Giardia lamblia* is a flagellate, both easy to identify when the trophozoites are visible in fecal preparations (NMS M&ID, 3rd Ed. p. 371–4)

16. The answer is D. Metronidazole is the drug of choice for symptomatic intestinal and extraintestinal amebiasis. Amphotericin B has been used with limited success in cases of primary meningoencephalitis; doxycycline is the drug of choice for *Balantidium coli;* iodoquinol is used for asymptomatic amebiasis; and quinacrine hydrochloride is effective against *Giardia*. (NMS M&ID, 3rd Ed. p. 365–8, 374)

17. The answer is E. The patient has meningitis caused by *Cryptococcus neoformans*. The result of the India ink test, which shows a small yeast surrounded by a large capsule, allows for the easy identification of this organism. *C. neoformans* is acquired by inhalation and can be isolated in large amounts from pigeon and chicken droppings. An epidemiological link between exposure to pigeon or chicken droppings and human infection has not been established. Blackbird roosts and bat guano are often loaded with *Histoplasma capsulatum*. Mexican pottery may harbor the arthrospores of *Coccidioides immitis*. Organic debris are the source of *Blastomyces dermatitidis*. (NMS M&ID, 3rd Ed. p. 348–354)

18. The answer is B. The large capsule of *Cryptococcus neoformans* is an effective antiphagocytic barrier. Once ingested, *C. neoformans* will be destroyed. The capsid or polysaccharide is as immunogenic as other microbial polysaccharides, and *C. neoformans* can be effectively treated with amphotericin B or, in milder cases, with fluconazole. (NMS M&ID, 3rd Ed. p. 348–9)

19. The answer is C. The symptoms presented by this child suggest pinworm infection, and the finding of small, oval embryonated eggs with one flattened side on a scotch tape applied to the perianal region confirms the diagnosis. The eggs of *Enterobius vermicularis* are small, light, and hardy and are easily aerosolized and ingested. All members of a household may be infected, even if only the youngest child is symptomatic. For that reason, some physicians recommend treating the whole family. (NMS M&ID, 3rd Ed. p. 389–90)

20. The answer is C. Mebendazole is the drug of choice for the most common nematode infections in the Western hemisphere, with the exception of strongyloidiasis, for which thiabendazole is the drug of choice. Pyrantel pamoate is effective for most of the same parasites that are treatable with mebendazole. (NMS M&ID, 3rd Ed. p. 389–94)

21. The answer is A. As indicated in question 20, mebendazole is the drug of choice. It disrupts microtubule formation and glucose transport, which are essential for pinworm survival. The closely related drug thiabendazole disrupts microtubules and inhibits fumarate reductase. Pyrantel, another effective antinematode drug, causes neuromuscular paralysis of the helminths, resulting in rapid expulsion from the gut. The drugs that inhibit glutathione-S-transferase (praziquantel) and uncouple oxidative phosphorylation (niclosamide) are used to treat cestode and nematode infections. (NMS M&ID, 3rd Ed. p. 368–9)

22. The answer is D. This HIV-positive patient presents with a bilateral interstitial pneumonia, and a broncho-alveolar lavage stained with methenamine-silver reveals cysts with multiple spores. The diagnosis of *Pneumocystis carinii* pneumonia is obvious, and the treatment of choice is intravenous administration of sulfamethoxazole-trimethoprim, a combination of drugs

that effectively blocks nucleotide synthesis. (NMS M&ID, 3rd Ed. p. 44, 48, 388, 425–6)

23. The answer is E. Patients with symptomatic HIV infection frequently have low granulocyte counts, because HIV infection interferes with normal hematopoiesis, and the function of those granulocytes that are present appears to be depressed. Both zidovudine (ZDV) and sulfamethoxazole-trimethoprim can cause bone marrow depression. This leads to very careful consideration of the advantages and disadvantages of giving ZDV to a patient that needs high doses of sulfamethoxazole-trimethoprim to treat a life-threatening condition. There are many other significant drug interactions that complicate the treatment of patients with AIDS, but in the case of ZDV and sulfamethoxazole-trimethoprim, bone marrow depression is the only consideration. (NMS M&ID, 3rd Ed. p. 513)

24. The answer is A. Most opportunistic fungal infections affect individuals with compromised cell-mediated immunity, reflecting the significance of cell-mediated mechanisms to eliminate fungi. AIDS is clearly a disease in which cell-mediated immunity is severely affected, and disseminated cryptococcal infections are among the opportunistic infections that affect AIDS patients. Note that *Aspergillus* infections are common in patients with chronic granulomatous disease and that neutropenia is often associated with candidiasis (although *Candida* will also prey on patients with AIDS and those with defects of cell-mediated immunity). (NMS M&ID, 3rd Ed. p. 357, 510)

25. The answer is D. Fluconazole, one of the azoles, is recommended for preventing recurrences of disseminated cryptococcal infection in immunocompromised individuals. Fluconazole is specially effective in preventing meningitis recurrences because it penetrates the CSF readily. Like all azoles, fluconazole blocks the conversion of lanosterol into 14-dimethyllanosterol, effectively blocking ergosterol synthesis. (NMS M&ID, 3rd Ed. p. 340–1, 349, 359) The other choices correspond to other antimycotic drugs that are not recommended for prophylaxis of cryptococcal meningitis recurrences, either because they are ineffective or because they are too toxic.

26. The answer is A. Because of its prevalence as a member of the normal intestinal flora and its role as an opportunistic agent, *Candida albicans* is the fungus most often isolated from patients with suspected mycoses. Whether infections with dermatophytes are more or less prevalent than infections with *C. albicans* is debatable, but very seldom do physicians submit skin scrapings for culture to characterize the responsible dermatophyte. (NMS M&ID, 3rd Ed. p. 347, 357)

27. The answer is B. The diagnosis of the different types of malaria is done by examining blood smears, looking for characteristic morphological features on the infected cells as well as morphological characteristics of *Plasmodia* trophozoites or gametocytes. The organisms are not cultured and the PIT test has been made up for this question. The duration of the latent period of the exoerythrocytic cycle is too variable and only applies to two species, *P. ovale* and *P. vivax*. Liver biopsies are not done for diagnosis of the species with persistent hepatic forms (hypnozoites) because the diagnosis can be made from examining blood films. (NMS M&ID, 3rd Ed. p. 382–4).

28. The answer is E. All of the mechanisms listed may account for recurrence or resistance to treatment of different parasitic infections, but not necessarily in the case of trypanosomiasis. Note also that the African trypanosomes do not infect red cells. The cause of relapses in African trypanosomiasis is a well-defined genetic mechanism that results in periodic changes in the major outer glycoprotein recognized by the immune system, and against which the protective immune response is directed. (NMS M&ID, 3rd Ed. p. 379)

29. The answer is C. There are three major targets for antifungal drugs: the enzymes involved in the different steps leading to ergosterol synthesis, the cell membrane, and the assembly of microtubules during cell division. Four of the most important groups of antimycotic agents block different steps in the ergosterol synthesis pathway. (NMS M&ID, 3rd Ed. p. 340–2)

30. The answer is B. Administering primaquine is contraindicated in individuals with glucose-6-phosphate dehydrogenase deficiency, because these patients develop acute hemolysis when given primaquine. The drug is otherwise indicated because of its effectiveness against liver forms. The darkening of the urine and acute renal failure are suggestive of massive hemolysis, leading to hemoglobinuria and acute tubular necrosis, due to hemoglobin toxicity. (NMS M&ID, 3rd Ed. p. 383–4; PAInfDis, 4th Ed. p. 831)

31. The answer is E. The hookworms (*Ancylostoma duodenale* and *Necator americanus*) cause multiple small bleeding lesions where they attach to the intestinal mucosa. Over a long period, this constant blood loss can result in an iron deficiency anemia. The only other realistic scenario leading to anemia as a consequence of a parasitic infection is lack of vitamin B_{12} from competition in its absorption by the parasite, which happens in patients infected with the fish tapeworm, *Diphyllobothrium latum*, particularly in Northern Europe. (NMS M&ID, 3rd Ed. p. 391–2, 399)

32. The answer is C. Most fungi are acquired from the environment, with some notable exceptions, such as *Candida albicans*, which is part of the normal intestinal flora and can be sexually transmitted, and the anthropophilic dermatophytes, such as *Epidermophyton floccosum*, which is transmitted from person to person via contaminated objects. (NMS M&ID, 3rd Ed. p. 343–4, 347)

33. The answer is B. *Trypanosoma cruzi*—the agent of South American trypanosomiasis or Chagas' disease—differs from the African trypanosomes in that it is found predominantly in tissues, where masses of amastigotes form intracellular pseudocysts. The C-shaped trypomastigotes are very difficult to visualize in the peripheral blood. The remaining choices correspond to signs or symptoms present at different stages of Chagas' disease. (NMS M&ID, 3rd Ed. p. 380–1)

34. The answer is A. The Duffy Fy^a and Fy^b blood group antigens serve as receptors for *Plasmodium vivax*, which does not infect Duffy-negative individuals, who do not express either one of the antigens. None of the other characteristics is unique to *P. vivax*, including the persistent infection of hepatic cells by hypnozoites, which is also the case in infections by *Plasmodium ovale*. (NMS M&ID, 3rd Ed. p. 382–4)

35. The answer is C. Coccidioidomycosis can mimic pulmonary tuberculosis, and the clinical picture as described does not allow a differential diagnosis between the two diseases. The fact that the patient is a farmer who resides on an area where *Coccidioides immitis* is prevalent in the soil, as well as the development of strong, persistent headaches, should raise the suspicion of coccidioidomycosis. *Cryptococcus neoformans* is also able to infect the CNS, but usually does not cause pulmonary symptoms such as those observed in this patient. *Histoplasma capsulatum* can cause pulmonary disease, but the area of geographic prevalence (the Mississippi-Ohio river basin) does not extend to Arizona. *Blastomyces* is found in the eastern half of North America and *Candida* does not usually cause pulmonary infections. (NMS M&ID, 3rd Ed. p. 348–9, 351–3)

36. The answer is A. Blastomycosis is acquired from organic debris, and individuals pursuing outdoors activities (such as farming) are at high risk. The ecological niche includes the eastern half of the United States. The clinical presentation includes cutaneous manifestations, such as skin ulcers, and respiratory symptoms, such as productive cough. *Histoplasma* and *Coccidioides* can also cause respiratory symptoms, but rarely cause skin lesions (particularly *Histoplasma*) and the ecological niches do not include the Southeast United States. *Cryptococcus* does not usually involve the skin, except in severely immunocompromised patients. *Sporothrix* causes a totally different disease, which may start with a cutaneous ulceration, but progresses subcutaneously, following the lymphatic vessels, until the infection reaches the regional lymph nodes. (NMS M&ID, 3rd Ed. p. 348–55)

37. The answer is B. Visceral larva migrans, caused by *Toxocara canis,* is characterized by fever, hepatomegaly, and eosinophilia in mild cases; and pulmonary infiltration with eosinophilia, endophthalmitis, gastrointestinal disturbances, splenomegaly, behavioral changes, seizures, and so forth in more severe cases. (NMS M&ID, 3rd Ed. p. 397–8)

38. The answer is E. Human carriers and domestic animals are rarely involved in the transmission of fungal diseases, with the exception of dermatophytic infections. Dried bird fecal material may be the source of *Histoplasma* or *Cryptococcus. Coccidioides* arthrospores can be carried by the wind and are acquired by inhalation. (NMS M&ID, 3rd Ed. p. 343, 349–51)

39. The answer is E. Direct microscopy of KOH preparations of affected nail scrapings is usually sufficient to confirm the diagnosis of tinea unguium infection. The species of dermatophyte may not be identified, but an adequate choice of antimycotic agent requires confirmation of the involvement of nails, rather than identification of the precise species involved. Thus, culture is not required. Exposure to UV light or serological assays are not used for diagnosis of tinea unguium. Itraconazole can be used for treatment, but rather than treating to make a diagnosis, the diagnosis should determine the treatment. (NMS M&ID, 3rd Ed. p. 339, 343–4)

40. The answer is C. The clinical vignette plus the histological findings are typical of chromomycosis. If the lesions are not very large and limited to the skin and subcutaneous region, surgical excision is the preferred treatment. If the disease is more extensive, amphotericin B or itraconazole may be tried. Itraconazole is also effective for treating sporotrichosis, replacing the classic treatment with oral potassium iodide. (NMS M&ID, 3rd Ed. p. 344–5)

41. The answer is A. As a rule, the best approach to confirm the diagnosis of any infectious disease is to positively identify the causative agent from a proper specimen, which in some cases may require culture and isolation, and in other cases may be achieved by other means. The India ink test is very useful in cases of cryptococcal meningitis, but cannot be used for the diagnosis of any other infection. KOH preparations of skin scrapings are only useful for the investigation of cutaneous, not systemic, mycoses. Serological tests and skin tests may be

useful in epidemiological studies but do not help when the objective is to diagnose an active systemic fungal infection. (NMS M&ID, 3rd Ed. p. 339–40)

42. The answer is D. Ingestion of undercooked meat containing cysts or ingestion of oocysts from cat feces are the two most important routes of infection for adults. In the United States ingestion of oocysts from cat feces is believed to be the most common way to acquire the disease. (NMS M&ID, 3rd Ed. p. 385–87)

43. The answer is D. *Anisakis* larvae are commonly found in both fish and squid. However, freezing is a very efficient way to destroy them, so even very poorly cooked seafood is safe if it has been previously frozen. Smoked fish, however, is not safe if it has only been lightly smoked. (NMS M&ID, 3rd Ed. p. 394–5)

44. The answer is B. Ingested *Ascaris* eggs hatch in the intestine and the larvae burrow through the intestinal wall and enter the lymphatic or portal circulation. Those entering the lymphatic circulation will reach the heart via the thoracic duct and from there will be transported to the lungs. Those entering the portal circulation will also reach the lung via the portal vein and the inferior vena cava. In the lungs the larvae molt twice, then enter the alveoli, and migrate to the intestine through the trachea, esophagus, and stomach. (NMS M&ID, 3rd Ed. p. 390–1)

45. The answer is D. The infective form of *Trichomonas vaginalis* is the trophozoite, which is very susceptible to desiccation. Therefore, transmission by fomites such as poorly washed and poorly dried towels, sponges, and so forth is possible, but rather unlikely and certainly much less frequent than transmission during intercourse. Fecal–oral transmission is a possibility with other parasites, but not with *T. vaginalis,* because its habitat does not include the intestine. (NMS M&ID, 3rd Ed. p. 376–7)

46. The answer is E. The easier explanation to rule out is the contamination of parenteral fluids, which are very carefully prepared and controlled to avoid this precise event. All other choices are likely to be contributory: the immaturity of the immune system, and the fact that any solution in the continuity of the skin represents a potential portal of entry for skin pathogens. However, the special prevalence of *Malassezia furfur* cannot be explained by these factors alone. The fact that parenteral nutrition fluids are very rich in long branch fatty acids, on the other hand, is significant, because those fatty acids are a specific growth requirement for *M. furfur.* (NMS M&ID, 3rd Ed. p. 358)

47. The answer is A. The clinical picture is suggestive of trichinellosis and would not fit in any of the other listed parasitic diseases. Anisakiasis and diphyllobothriasis, besides having different presentations, are contracted by eating fish from northern latitudes, not tropical fish. Bear meat, on the other hand, very frequently harbors *Trichinella* larvae, and can be the source of infection for hunters who do not cook the meat adequately. (NMS M&ID, 3rd Ed. p. 390–4, 399)

48. The answer is D. In a symptomatic case of trichinellosis, the parasite larvae are encysted in striated muscle cells, so examination of stool material will not demonstrate the parasite. A CBC and differential may demonstrate eosinophilia, but several other parasitic infections may cause the same finding. The finding of anti-*Trichinella* antibodies can help establish a tentative diagnosis, but confirmation is only possible by visualizing the parasite in a muscle biopsy (NMS M&ID, 3rd Ed. p. 392–4).

49. The answer is A. The picture reproduces a perfect specimen of *Aspergillus,* a filamentous fungus, with septated hyphae that branch at 45° angles. *Aspergillus* often infects healed cavities of patients with inactive tuberculosis. *Mucor* and *Rhizopus* are also filamentous fungi, but they are not septated. *Nocardia* is a filamentous bacteria, which is best revealed with an acid-fast stain. *Malassezia furfur* causes tinea versicolor and its typical appearance is described as "spaghetti and meatballs," corresponding to intertwined hyphae and budding yeasts. (NMS M&ID, 3rd Ed. p. 189–91, 344–6)

50. The answer is E. The presentation and histological findings (broad, nonseptated hyphae) are typical of zygomycosis, which is caused by three genera of fungi (*Rhizopus, Mucor,* and *Absidia*) with worldwide distribution. The association with uncontrolled diabetes is remarkable and is one of the most important elements that may allow early diagnosis. (NMS M&ID, 3rd Ed. p. 345–6).

TEST 5

Infectious Diseases

Test 5

Infectious Diseases

LIST OF COMMON ABBREVIATIONS

AIDS	acquired immunodeficiency syndrome	HSV	herpes simplex virus
CAMP	Christie-Atkins-and-Munch-Peterson [test]	HTLV	human lymphotropic virus
CBC	complete blood count	Ig	immunoglobulin
CMV	cytomegalovirus	IL	interleukin
CSF	cerebrospinal fluid	KOH	potassium hydroxide
DNA	deoxyribonucleic acid	MHC	major histocompatibility complex
HB_cAg	hepatitis B core antigen	MRI	magnetic resonance imaging
HB_sAg	hepatitis B surface antigen	RNA	ribonucleic acid
HBV	hepatitis B virus; also HAV, HCV, HDV, HEV	TNF	tumor necrosis factor
HIV	human immunodeficiency virus	WBC	white blood cell

LIST OF BACTERIA

E. coli   *Escherichia coli*
H. pylori   *Helicobacter pylori*

Directions: (Items 1–73) Each of the numbered items or incomplete statements in this section is followed by answers or by completions of the statement. Select the ONE lettered answer or completion that is BEST in each case.

QUESTIONS 1–3

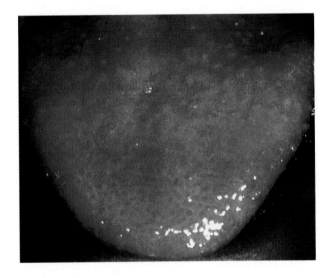

A 4-year-old boy is brought to the emergency department because he had a high fever after complaining of a sore throat.

Vital signs:

temperature: 40.5°C
respiratory rate: 30/minute
pulse: 120/minute
blood pressure: 120/70 mmHg.

Physical examination showed an abnormal tongue (see the figure) and a faintly erythematous and patchy rash in the trunk which, at touch, felt like sandpaper, and blanches with pressure. Remaining physical examination is within normal limits.

1. The virulence factor responsible for this patient's enanthema and exanthem is encoded by a

(A) Bacterial chromosomal gene
(B) Gene carried by a lysogenic phage
(C) Gene carried by a generalized transducing phage
(D) Specific virulence plasmid
(E) Transposon

2. The patient's fever is caused by

(A) A bacterial exotoxin
(B) Bacterial lipopolysaccharide
(C) Increased metabolic rate
(D) Loss of fluids
(E) M protein

3. The infection is best treated with

(A) A third-generation cephalosporin
(B) Erythromycin
(C) Penicillin G
(D) Supportive therapy (antipyretics, fluids)
(E) Vancomycin

QUESTIONS 4–5

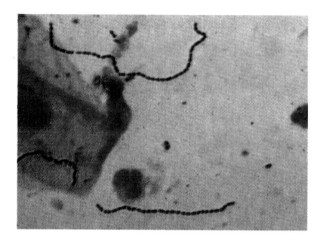

After prolonged labor, a male baby is born with a low Apgar score. His temperature is 37.2°C; he is tachycardic, tachypneic, and lethargic. He develops seizures, and a CSF sample reveals high protein, low sugar, and abundant neutrophils. A Gram stain reveals the organisms shown in the figure, which after culture are found to be β-hemolytic, bacitracin-resistant, and positive in the CAMP test.

4. This organism is most likely

(A) Group A *Streptococcus*
(B) Group B *Streptococcus*
(C) *Listeria monocytogenes*
(D) *Staphylococcus albus*
(E) *Neisseria meningitidis*

5. The antimicrobial of choice to treat this patient is

(A) Penicillin G
(B) Vancomycin
(C) Doxycycline
(D) Metronidazole
(E) Erythromycin

QUESTIONS 6–7

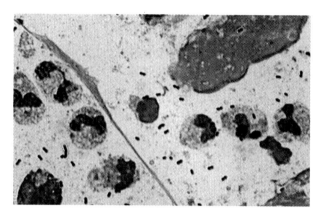

A 4-year-old child with a history of recurrent pulmonary infections has been brought to the emergency department in obvious respiratory distress. The figure reproduces a Gram stain of the sputum.

6. Which of the following tests would best identify the microorganism most likely involved in this patient's infection?

(A) Bacitracin sensitivity
(B) Bile solubility
(C) Hemolysis pattern
(D) Indole fermentation
(E) Oxidase activity

7. Which of the following drugs would be adequate for initial treatment while waiting for the child's antibiotic sensitivity report to arrive?

(A) Ceftriaxone
(B) Chloramphenicol
(C) Gentamicin
(D) Penicillin G
(E) Streptomycin

QUESTIONS 8–11

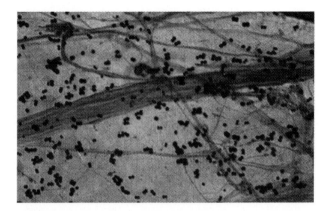

A 3-month-old boy is brought to the emergency department in respiratory difficulty. An emergency radiograph of the thorax shows diffuse bilateral infiltrates, and the organism in the figure is visualized on a Gram stain of a smear of the sediment of a bronchial aspirate. Physical examination revealed an oozing lesion on the scalp and an enlarged lymph node in the occipital region. A needle aspirate of the lymph node was obtained and revealed abundant neutrophils with intracellular cocci.

8. This disease is the result of the

(A) Deficient antibody response to common organisms
(B) Inability of lysosomes to fuse with phagosomes
(C) Lack of assembly of a functional oxidase on the phagosome membrane
(D) Lack of terminal complement components
(E) Severe depletion of CD4+ T lymphocytes

9. The genetic defect most commonly found in this disease is a deletion or mutation of the

(A) Bruton's tyrosine kinase gene
(B) Cytochrome B heavy chain gene
(C) Lysozyme gene
(D) Nitric synthetase gene
(E) Zymosan-activated plasma (ZAP) kinase gene

10. After his current pulmonary infection is treated, this child should be placed on prophylactic therapy with

(A) Fluconazole
(B) Gamma globulin
(C) Sulfamethoxazole-trimethoprim
(D) Tetracycline
(E) Vancomycin

11. Which one of the following compounds has been found to reduce the frequency of infections that affect patients with this disease?

(A) Ascorbic acid
(B) Granulocyte-macrophage colony-stimulating factor
(C) Interferon-γ
(D) IL-12
(E) IL-2

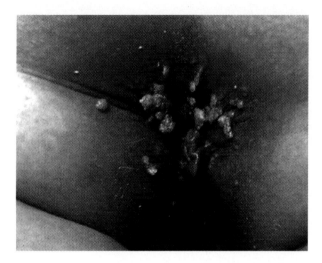

12. Which one of the following viruses is most likely to be recovered from the perianal lesions shown in the figure?

(A) HSV, type 1
(B) HSV, type 2
(C) Human papilloma virus 6 or 11
(D) Human papilloma virus 16 or 18
(E) Human herpesvirus 8

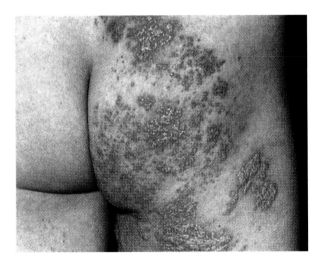

13. A 56-year-old woman under treatment for inoperable breast cancer develops the rash shown in the figure. Cytological examination of scrapings from the base of one of the vesicles reveals cells with intranuclear inclusions. The virus responsible for these lesions can be best described as

    (A) An enveloped, helical, DNA virus
    (B) An enveloped, helical, RNA virus
    (C) An enveloped, icosahedral, DNA virus
    (D) A naked, helical, RNA virus
    (E) A naked, icosahedral, DNA virus

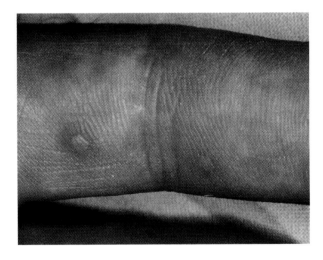

14. A child presents with the lesions shown in the figure and multiple vesicular eruptions on the hard palate. A closely related infectious agent is most likely to also cause

    (A) Cervical carcinoma
    (B) Genital warts
    (C) Infantile diarrhea
    (D) Myocarditis
    (E) Pleurodynia

QUESTIONS 15–16

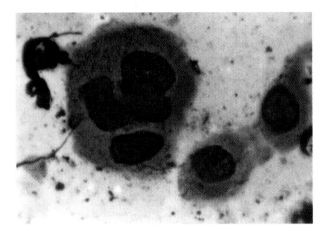

A 66-year-old woman receiving chemotherapy for inoperable breast cancer develops a painful vesicular hemorrhagic rash in her right anterior chest. Cytological examination of scrapings from the base of one of the vesicles reveals the cells shown in the figure.

15. To confirm the diagnosis of this patient's disease you should

    (A) Ask for an HIV viral load
    (B) Culture the scrapings from the base of another vesicle
    (C) Order a special stain for Guarnieri bodies
    (D) Perform a direct immunofluorescence study on the scrapings using enzyme-labeled anti-HSV 1 and 2 antibodies
    (E) Test the vesicular fluid for Coxsackievirus antigens

16. In addition to the illustrated cytopathic effect, the virus responsible for these lesions may cause

    (A) B cell immortalization
    (B) Expression of T antigens on the infected cell membrane
    (C) Intracytoplasmic inclusion bodies
    (D) Intranuclear inclusion bodies
    (E) Rapid lysis of infected cells

QUESTIONS 17–18

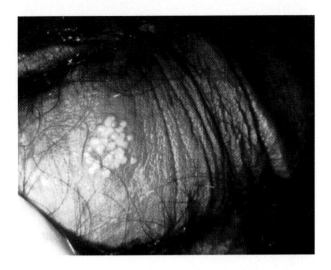

A sexually active 22-year-old man presents to the sexually transmitted disease (STD) clinic with the lesions shown in the figure. A scraping of the base of one of the vesicles shows multinucleated giant cells. He explains that he had a similar eruption in the same area 2 months earlier.

17. The recurrent nature of this patient's lesions is a consequence of

- (A) Variation of the antigenic make-up of the causative agent
- (B) Lack of immunogenicity of the responsible infectious agent
- (C) A second infection with a similar virus with a different serotype
- (D) Rapid development of resistance to antiviral agents
- (E) Reactivation of a latent infection in a sensory ganglion

18. The best preventive measure to avoid transmitting this disease to his sexual partners is to

- (A) Apply topical famciclovir before intercourse
- (B) Immunize all noninfected contacts
- (C) Administer prophylactic acyclovir to the patient and his partner(s)
- (D) Treat all lesions with interferon-α
- (E) Use barrier contraceptives

QUESTIONS 19–20

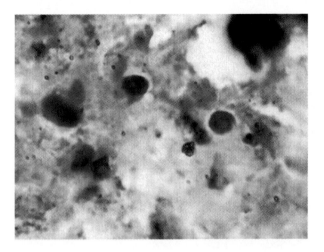

An outbreak of infectious diarrhea affected 25 patients in a teaching hospital in Minneapolis, Minnesota. The patients affected included 5 premature babies, 9 patients treated for a variety of malignancies, 8 HIV-positive patients, and 3 geriatric patients over 80 years old. In 17 of the patients the organisms shown in the figure were detected in formalin-fixed stool samples stained with Kinyoun's stain.

19. The infectious agent responsible for the outbreak is most likely

- (A) *Entamoeba histolytica*
- (B) *Giardia lamblia*
- (C) *Cryptosporidium parvum*
- (D) *Cyclospora cayetanensis*
- (E) *Isospora belli*

20. The most likely source for this organism is

- (A) Berries
- (B) Contaminated meat
- (C) Fresh salads
- (D) Hands of health care practitioners
- (E) Water supply

QUESTIONS 21–22

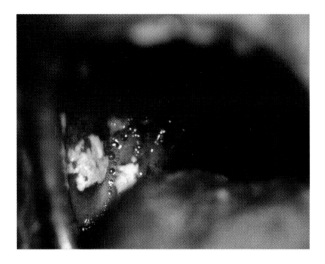

A 6-year-old boy receiving chemotherapy for acute lymphoblastic leukemia develops a persistent fever that is not affected by administration of broad-spectrum antibiotics. Physical examination shows the lesions reproduced in the figure and an erythematous rash in the perineal region. A CBC shows leukopenia (1000 leukocytes/mm^3, 70% lymphocytes with many blastic forms, 20% neutrophils, 8% monocytes, 2% basophils).

21. This patient may have a systemic infection caused by

(A) *Aspergillus fumigatus*
(B) *Candida albicans*
(C) *Cryptococcus neoformans*
(D) *Histoplasma capsulatum*
(E) *Rhizopus* species

22. To confirm the diagnosis, which of the following should be ordered?

(A) A KOH preparation of a smear of the white exudate in the oral mucosa
(B) Blood cultures in Sabouraud's agar
(C) Fecal cultures in MacConkey and blood agars
(D) Fecal cultures in Sabouraud's agar
(E) Serological tests for *Candida albicans*

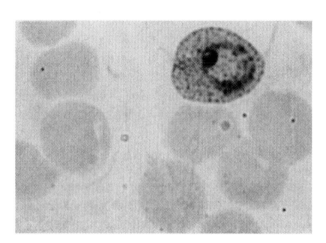

23. A 27-year-old white man sought medical attention because of recurrent fever for the past 3 weeks, after he returned from a trip to the forests of Venezuela. Laboratory work-up reveals anemia, increased conjugated and total bilirubin, decreased haptoglobin, and traces of hemoglobin in the urine. The blood smear reveals the abnormalities shown in the figure. This patient is most likely infected by

(A) *Babesia microti*
(B) *Leishmania tropica*
(C) *Plasmodium falciparum*
(D) *Plasmodium vivax*
(E) *Trypanosoma cruzi*

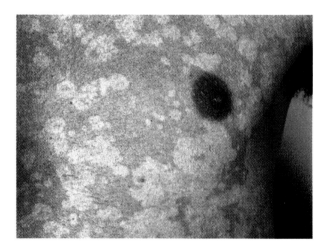

24. The skin lesions shown in the figure are most likely the consequence of an infection caused by

(A) *Borrelia burgdorferi*
(B) Group A *Streptococcus*
(C) *Malassezia furfur*
(D) Measles virus
(E) Mycobacterium leprae

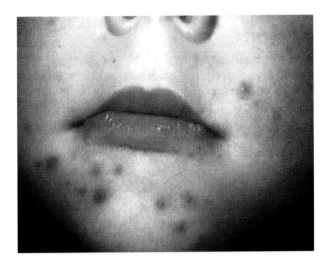

25. A 5-year-old girl presents with fever (103°F) and a rash that started in the trunk and has spread to the face (see the figure). This child most likely has an infection caused by

(A) Coxsackie A virus
(B) HSV
(C) Measles virus
(D) *Streptococcus pyogenes*
(E) Varicella-zoster virus

QUESTIONS 26–27

A 36-year-old woman with a history of drug abuse and hepatitis C presents complaining of progressive tiredness, ankle swelling and eye puffiness, migratory joint pains predominantly affecting the knees and elbows, and a nonblanching maculopapular rash over her lower extremities.

26. Which of the following findings would be most helpful in explaining this patient's symptoms?

(A) Elevated bilirubin
(B) Granular casts in the urine
(C) Mixed cryoglobulinemia
(D) Positive rheumatoid factor
(E) Proteinuria

27. What type of antiviral agent could be therapeutically useful in this patient?

(A) A DNA synthesis inhibitor
(B) A protease inhibitor
(C) A protein synthesis inhibitor
(D) A reverse transcriptase inhibitor
(E) An RNA polymerase inhibitor

28. A 32-year-old male HBV carrier with a history of intravenous drug abuse presents in the emergency department after collapsing in the street. He is deeply jaundiced, and has a fever of 101°F. He reports that he has had 2 other episodes of jaundice in the past 14 months for which he did not seek medical attention. He states that this is the worst he has ever felt and admits to current intravenous drug use. The most likely diagnosis is superinfection with

(A) HAV
(B) HBV
(C) HDV
(D) HEV
(E) HIV

29. A pregnant woman presents for prenatal care. She says she had been sick 3 years before with jaundice that was accompanied by intestinal upset, and was followed by joint pains and a rash that affected mostly her legs and slowly subsided. She has felt well in the last 2 years. The possibility that this woman may still be harboring the infectious agent that caused her disease and that she could transmit it to her baby is considered. Which laboratory test would be the most important to order?

(A) Blood test for malaria
(B) HBV surface antigen
(C) HIV serologies
(D) IgM antibody to HB$_c$ Ag
(E) Quantitation of HAV IgM antibody

30. A 20-year-old man presents with a penile lesion that is crateriform, moist, and peripherally indurated. Questioning the patient revealed that this lesion has been present for about 10 days, and is not noticeably painful. Which test would you order to investigate whether this patient may have syphilis?

(A) Blood cultures
(B) Culture of the exudate
(C) Gram stain of the exudate
(D) Microhemagglutination *Treponema pallidum* test (MHA-TP)
(E) Venereal Disease Research Laboratory (VDRL) test

QUESTIONS 31–32

A 24-year-old, sexually active woman was well until 3 days ago when she woke up feeling slightly nauseated. On the same day she felt pain and tenderness in her lower abdomen while jogging. She had to stop exercising and get a ride home. The pain was sharp in nature and didn't radiate. She took 4 ibuprofen pills, which relieved the pain slightly, but over the next 3 days the pain and nausea increased in intensity. She denies any vomiting, diarrhea, or change in bowel habits. She reports slight burning on urination, but no increased frequency or urgency. Vital signs: temperature 102°F; respiratory movements 21/minute; pulse 78/minute; blood pressure (sitting) 128/70. On physical examination she appears uncomfortable, leaning forward on the edge of the chair. Abdominal palpation shows liver edge 2 cm below the rib margin, and it is nontender. There is bilateral lower quadrant tenderness, which is worse on the right. No masses felt. Pelvic examination reveals positive cervical motion tenderness, scanty cervical mucopurulent discharge, and bilateral adnexal tenderness, which is worse on the right side.

31. The treatment of this disease has to take into consideration that

(A) Emergency surgery is the indicated approach for this patient
(B) Several bacteria with different antibiotic susceptibilities may be involved
(C) The decision about treatment should wait until the results of cervical exudate cultures become available
(D) The patient may be at risk for developing septic shock
(E) The patient may be infected by organisms secreting potent superantigens

32. A most likely complication for this patient's condition is

(A) Infertility
(B) Kidney insufficiency
(C) Liver cirrhosis
(D) Peritoneal perforation
(E) Sepsis

33. On a global scale, which one of the following factors is likely to have a stronger impact on the risk of contracting HIV infection?

(A) Age
(B) Gender
(C) Race
(D) Sexual preference
(E) Socioeconomic status

34. With the introduction of a more effective vaccine, which organism has markedly decreased in frequency as the cause of systemic infections in infants in the last few years?

(A) *Bordetella pertussis*
(B) *Haemophilus influenzae*
(C) HBV
(D) *Neisseria meningitidis*
(E) *Streptococcus pneumoniae*

QUESTIONS 35–36

The patient is a 40-year-old mother of 4 children who was re-admitted to the hospital with general complaints of fever (39°C), malaise, anorexia, and flank pain. She had been released from the hospital about 3 days before this last admission, after removal of an ovarian cyst. Her bladder had been catheterized during her last admission and review of her records showed that she had fever 24 hours after surgery. She was treated with ampicillin. A urine specimen obtained after re-admission was found to contain pus cells and casts. A urine culture yielded colonies of an oxidase-positive, gram-negative rod that released a green diffusible pigment.

35. This is likely to be a case of

(A) Bacteremia
(B) Cystitis
(C) Glomerulonephritis
(D) Pyelonephritis
(E) Urethritis

36. The agent that caused this condition is likely to be

(A) *E. coli*
(B) *Klebsiella pneumoniae*
(C) *Proteus mirabilis*
(D) *Pseudomonas aeruginosa*
(E) *Streptococcus viridans*

QUESTIONS 37–38

A veterinarian complaining of malaise and yellowing of sclera seeks medical attention. Physical examination confirms the existence of hepatomegaly and jaundice. Serologies for hepatitis A and B and blood cultures are negative. Renal function tests suggest moderate impairment of tubular function. Serum creatinine kinase is elevated.

37. The most likely diagnosis is

(A) Hepatitis E
(B) Leptospirosis
(C) Lyme disease
(D) Malaria
(E) Relapsing fever

38. A most likely source of this patient's infection was

(A) Blood or blood products from an infected animal
(B) Contaminated drinking water
(C) Dog urine
(D) Mosquito bite
(E) Tick bite

39. A 2-year-old child with acute bronchopneumonia is admitted through the emergency department. A bronchial aspirate is collected for direct examination and cultures. On direct examination, the finding of large multinucleated cellular clumps is reported. To further clarify the diagnosis while this child is in the emergency department, you could send a nasopharyngeal swab to the laboratory and order

(A) Bacterial cultures
(B) Cold agglutinin titer
(C) Gram stain and acid-fast stain
(D) Rapid test for respiratory syncytial virus
(E) Viral cultures for respiratory syncytial virus and parainfluenza virus

QUESTIONS 40–41

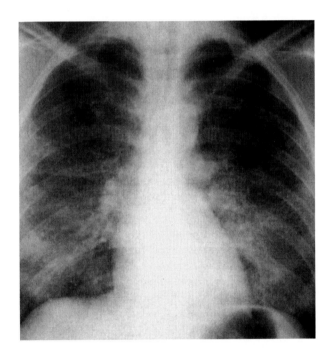

An HIV-positive individual is seen at the emergency department with shortness of breath and cyanosis. The chest radiograph is shown in the figure.

40. The most likely cause for this patient's lung infection is

(A) *Chlamydia psittaci*
(B) CMV
(C) HSV, type 1
(D) *Klebsiella pneumoniae*
(E) *Pneumocystis carinii*

41. Treatment of this condition should involve administering

(A) Acyclovir
(B) Ceftriaxone and gentamicin
(C) Doxycycline
(D) Ganciclovir
(E) Trimethoprim-sulfamethoxazole

QUESTIONS 42–43

A 31-year-old woman, pregnant for 2 months, is found to be HIV-positive during prenatal checking. Her CD4 count is 600/μL and the viral load was measured at 30,000/μL.

42. The most adequate course of action is to

(A) Follow the CD4 counts and viral loads every 3 months, withholding therapy until the CD4 count drops below 400/mm³
(B) Start treatment with a combination of zidovudine, a second reverse transcriptase inhibitor, and a protease inhibitor after the 14th week of gestation
(C) Start treatment with zidovudine at week 14 and add additional antiretrovirals if the viral load fails to decrease
(D) Start treatment with zidovudine at week 14 and maintain this regimen until delivery

43. If proper therapeutic measures are adopted, the risk of fetal infection is

(A) 60%–70%
(B) 50%–60%
(C) 25%–50%
(D) 10%–25%
(E) less than 10%

44. The risk of fetal infection with HIV is greater

(A) After birth, if the baby is breast-fed
(B) During the first trimester of pregnancy
(C) During the third trimester of pregnancy
(D) In the perinatal period

45. A 28-year-old woman seeks medical attention at the emergency department because she is having an abnormally prolonged and intense menstrual period. Besides bleeding profusely she has had fever up to 103°F, has felt very tired and sleepy, and has had progressively severe diarrhea, which in the last day has been laced with blood. Physical examination shows she is tachycardic, tachypneic, with cold, damp skin, and a blood pressure of 80/40. Faint, diffuse erythema is noted on the neck and upper half of the thorax. The woman is admitted, bacteriological cultures are ordered, and both supportive therapy and antibiotics are started. Many of her symptoms are likely to result from the release by the causative agent of a toxin that causes

(A) Dissolution of lipid bilayer membranes
(B) Epidermolysis
(C) Hemolysis
(D) Massive release of pro-inflammatory cytokines
(E) Persistent activation of adenyl cyclase in mucosal cells

46. Which of the following infections is most likely to be classified as opportunistic?

(A) Brucellosis in a veterinarian
(B) *E. coli* bacteremia in a leukemic patient receiving chemotherapy
(C) Giardiasis in a nursery staff member
(D) *H. pylori* infection in a young adult of Mediterranean descent
(E) Pulmonary tuberculosis in a young medicine resident

47. A 32-year-old man is admitted with a tentative diagnosis of viral encephalitis. There is no history of exposure to mosquitoes in the previous couple of weeks and there is no known outbreak of viral encephalitis in the community. A needle biopsy of the frontal lobe of the brain is inconclusive. An MRI of the brain is compatible with viral encephalitis. The most important intervention in this patient is to

(A) Keep the patient in the hospital for a few more days under close observation
(B) Order serologies for the most common agents of viral encephalitis
(C) Perform a spinal tap and send CSF for direct examination and culture
(D) Start a third-generation cephalosporin intravenous line immediately
(E) Start treatment with acyclovir immediately

QUESTIONS 48–49

A 32-year-old migrant worker who recently arrived from South America is hospitalized for treatment of recurrent fever and severe headaches and back aches. A CBC with differential shows mild anemia and slight leukocytosis, with predominance of lymphocytes. CSF examination is negative. A search for eggs and parasites in the feces is negative. A thick blood smear for malaria parasites is also negative. Speaking through an interpreter, he indicates that he worked as a sheep herdsman before crossing the border looking for work.

48. This is most likely a case of

(A) Amebiasis
(B) Brucellosis
(C) Salmonellosis
(D) South American trypanosomiasis
(E) Viral encephalitis

49. The disease was most likely acquired by

(A) Ingesting food contaminated by an infected food handler
(B) Ingesting unpasteurized milk or cheese
(C) Triatomine bug bite
(D) Mosquito bite
(E) Sexual intercourse

50. To evaluate the effectiveness of antiretroviral treatment in an HIV-infected patient, which is the preferred assay?

(A) CD4+ T cell count
(B) Determining the proportion of infected cells in a lymph node biopsy
(C) Quantitative assay of plasma viral RNA by polymerase chain reaction
(D) Quantitative assay of soluble viral antigens in the plasma
(E) Viral culture of the peripheral blood

51. Which of the following immunizations is recommended for administration to the newborn **immediately** after birth?

(A) Conjugated *Haemophilus influenzae* (HiB) vaccine
(B) Diphtheria-tetanus-acellular pertussis (DTaP) vaccine
(C) Hepatitis B vaccine
(D) Inactivated polio vaccine
(E) Measles-mumps-rubella (MMR) vaccine

52. A 4-day-old female infant is brought to the emergency department because of inconsolable crying, refusal to feed, and occasional vomiting which began within the past 6 hours. The mother's pregnancy had been uncomplicated and her delivery was uneventful. The child had no problems as a newborn and was discharged with her mother 36 hours after delivery. On examination she appeared listless but was irritable when handled or moved. Her breathing was shallow and her respiratory rate was 68/minute. Her temperature was 36.2°C, her pulse was 160/minute, and her blood pressure was 72/54 mm Hg. She had no rash but her hands and feet were pale, blotchy, and cool to the touch. Her chest radiograph was normal. A CBC revealed a white count of 12,400 WBC/mm^3 with a left shift (61% polymorphonuclear leukocytes with 10% band forms). Of the following measures and concerns, which one would you give the lowest priority in this infant?

- (A) Collect CSF for Gram stain and cultures as soon as possible
- (B) Evaluate possible increase of intracranial pressure
- (C) Initiate empiric antibiotherapy
- (D) Order blood cultures for bacteria
- (E) Order enteroviral cultures of the CSF

53. A 43-year-old woman is brought to the emergency department after wandering out in apparent confusion from the scene of a minor traffic accident for which she was responsible. Screens for alcohol and drugs were negative. The MRI showed abnormal areas of hyperintensity disseminated through the white matter of both hemispheres. Serologies for CMV and HIV were negative. IgG antitoxoplasma antibodies were positive in serum. Antimeasles hemagglutinin antibody titers were 640 in serum and 5120 in CSF. This patient is likely to be suffering from

- (A) Cerebral toxoplasmosis
- (B) Creutzfeldt-Jakob disease
- (C) Herpes encephalitis
- (D) Multiple sclerosis
- (E) Subacute sclerosing panencephalitis

QUESTIONS 54–55

A 50-year-old woman is admitted to the emergency department with profuse, watery diarrhea in November 1991. She had just returned from Lima, Peru, and started to feel sick during the last leg of her trip. She flew from Lima to Miami and several passengers on the same flight suffered from similar symptoms. The food, which included fresh garden salad, shrimp cocktail, grilled salmon, roast beef, and éclairs was boarded at the flight's origin.

54. Which foodstuff was most likely the source of this patient's infection?

- (A) Fresh garden salad
- (B) Shrimp cocktail
- (C) Grilled salmon
- (D) Roast beef
- (E) Éclairs

55. The most important measure to take in this patient is to

- (A) Administer antidiarrheal medications
- (B) Administer fluids and electrolytes
- (C) Collect blood and fecal material for culture
- (D) Collect fecal material for enterotoxin screening
- (E) Initiate antimicrobial therapy

56. A 28-year-old Mexican migrant worker is seen in the emergency department complaining of abdominal cramps and diarrhea. He is found to be febrile. Stool examination shows soft and scant fecal material with abundant mucus and no visible blood. A quick test for occult blood is positive. A fecal smear is stained with Wright's stain and shows abundant leukocytes. Of the following diagnostic tests, which one would you give the lowest priority?

- (A) Fecal cultures for *E. coli*
- (B) Fecal cultures for Norwalk virus
- (C) Fecal cultures for *Salmonella*
- (D) Fecal cultures for *Shigella*
- (E) Search for eggs and parasites (O&P) in the feces

QUESTIONS 57–58

A 20-year-old college student develops fever, fatigue, sore throat, and cervical lymphadenopathy about a month after Christmas vacation. He is seen at the student health center and found to have a pharyngitis with enlarged tonsils and palatal petechiae; cervical, axillary, and inguinal lymphadenopathy; and hepatosplenomegaly. Laboratory tests show normal red cell count and hemoglobin, and a positive test for heterophile hemagglutinins.

57. The agent most likely to be responsible for this disease is

- (A) CMV
- (B) Epstein-Barr virus
- (C) Group A *Streptococcus*
- (D) *Mycoplasma hominis*
- (E) *Neisseria gonorrhoeae*

58. The best treatment for this patient is

(A) Acyclovir

(B) Ceftriaxone

(C) Doxycycline

(D) Penicillin G

(E) Supportive measures

QUESTIONS 59–60

A 26-year-old Mexican exchange student is referred to the university hospital for investigation of a persistent abdominal pain and weight loss. He indicates that his current symptoms were preceded by chronic, intermittent, bloody diarrhea for about 1 year preceding his move to the United States. Physical examination reveals hepatomegaly, and the liver is tender at palpation. The CBC and differential show leukocytosis (13,000/μL) with 65% neutrophils. An abdominal ultrasound reveals a cavitary lesion in the liver.

59. This patient's condition is most likely caused by

(A) *Entamoeba histolytica*

(B) *Fasciola hepatica*

(C) *Salmonella enteritidis*

(D) *Schistosoma mansoni*

(E) *Shigella sonnei*

60. The virulence of the responsible organism is related to the secretion of

(A) Cysteine protease

(B) Intercellular spread protein

(C) Invasin

(D) Shiga-like toxin

(E) Vacuolating cytotoxin

61. A 75-year-old woman from a rural area of the southeast is admitted because of complications following a farm accident, which resulted in an open fracture of her leg. She sought medical attention at a local clinic, where her fracture was immobilized. She had surgery 2 days later but has now developed pharyngeal spasms when she tries to swallow and general rigidity of all muscles. When stimulated by loud noises, she suffers from generalized muscle spasms, opisthotonos, and risus sardonicus. The most effective and least costly method for prevention of this disease is

(A) Active immunization immediately after the injury

(B) Administration of antibiotics immediately after the injury

(C) Cleaning and débriding the wound immediately after injury

(D) Immunization at regular intervals

(E) Passive immunization immediately after the injury

62. Which of the following infections is transmitted by ticks?

(A) Bartonellosis

(B) Dengue

(C) Ehrlichiosis

(D) Leishmaniasis

(E) Typhus

63. Which of the following infections of the nervous system is caused by a retrovirus?

(A) Bovine spongiform encephalopathy

(B) Creutzfeldt-Jakob disease

(C) Kuru

(D) Progressive multifocal encephalopathy

(E) Progressive spastic paraparesis

64. Which of the following infectious agents has been proven to stimulate the synthesis of antibodies that are cross-reactive with neuron gangliosides?

(A) *Bordetella pertussis*

(B) *Campylobacter jejuni*

(C) Measles virus

(D) Parainfluenza virus

(E) Varicella-zoster virus

65. An 18-month-old baby girl presented to the emergency department with fever and a diffuse rash. Her temperature was 40°C, and her heart rate was 180/minute. Physical examination showed a rash, more pronounced in the trunk, with both macular and vesicular lesions. Four vesicular lesions could be seen in the soft palate. The remainder of the physical examination was unremarkable. The chest radiograph was clear; CBC with differential showed a total WBC count of 9000 with normal differential. This child most likely has

(A) Chickenpox

(B) Herpangina

(C) Measles

(D) Roseola infantum

(E) Scarlet fever

QUESTIONS 66–67

A healthy 4-year-old girl is taken to her pediatrician by a mother concerned because over the period of a week the child lost her appetite, complained of pains in her legs and back, became apathetic, and developed a high fever, at which time her eyes appeared to have a yellow discoloration. On physical examination, the child was lethargic but awake. Mild jaundice was noted, and some tenderness was apparent over the liver. Her body temperature was 100.1°F, and the pulse rate 80/minute. The child's mother mentions that several other children at the same day-care center had recently had similar symptoms and that she gave aspirin to the child the day before the doctor's appointment, to lower her temperature.

66. Your preliminary diagnosis in this case is

(A) CMV infection
(B) Hepatitis A
(C) Hepatitis E
(D) Leptospirosis
(E) Reye's syndrome

67. The most likely evolution for this patient is

(A) Chronic disease with manifestations similar to serum sickness
(B) Clinical improvement but the patient remains chronically infected
(C) Complete recovery
(D) Progression to coma, with a 10%–40% risk of death
(E) Prolonged convalescence with risk of developing liver failure

68. Which of the following infections is considered pathognomonic for AIDS?

(A) Cryptococcal meningitis
(B) Esophageal candidiasis
(C) Pulmonary histoplasmosis
(D) *Salmonella* bacteremia
(E) Vaginal candidiasis

69. Immunoprophylaxis can prevent which of these malignancies?

(A) Adult T cell leukemia
(B) Bladder carcinoma
(C) Burkitt's lymphoma
(D) Cervical carcinoma
(E) Hepatoma

70. Which congenital infection should be investigated in a newborn showing microcephaly, cerebral calcifications, and chorioretinitis?

(A) CMV
(B) Herpes simplex
(C) Rubella
(D) Syphilis
(E) Toxoplasmosis

71. On a global scale, a major cause of infantile morbidity and mortality are infections with

(A) *Campylobacter jejuni*
(B) *E. coli* O157:H7
(C) *Giardia lamblia*
(D) Norwalk virus
(E) Rotavirus

QUESTIONS 72–73

An unconscious 20-year-old man was transported to the emergency department. According to friend he had been drinking heavily and passed out in a fraternity house, where he may have been unconscious for several hours before the emergency medical service was called. There was dry vomit on his clothes. On physical examination the patient remained stuporous and unable to respond to commands, had a temperature of 103°F, and a fetid odor on his breath. Thoracic examination revealed dullness to percussion and absent breath sounds over the right posterior midlung field. The remaining physical examination was unremarkable.

72. This patient's lung infection is most likely a result of

(A) Aspiration of anaerobes from the oral cavity
(B) Aspiration of bacteria from the lower gastrointestinal tract
(C) Colonization of translocated intestinal bacteria
(D) Depressed immunity facilitating infection by opportunistic bacteria
(E) Depressed ventilatory function

73. Initial treatment of this patient should include the antibiotic

(A) Ceftriaxone
(B) Ciprofloxacin
(C) Clindamycin
(D) Penicillin G
(E) Vancomycin

Directions: (Items 74–75) Each of the numbered items or incomplete statements in this section is negatively phrased, as indicated by a capitalized word such as NOT, LEAST, or EXCEPT. Select the ONE lettered answer or completion that is BEST in each case.

74. A 36-year-old man presents because of fever and headache. He was well until 3 weeks earlier when he began to have daily generalized headaches. Initially they were relieved by aspirin, but after 2 weeks the headaches were more severe, and he began to have daily fever. Physical examination reveals an ill-appearing man with an oral temperature of 101°F (38.3°C). Nuchal rigidity is noted; the rest of the examination is normal. Lumbar puncture reveals clear spinal fluid with an opening pressure of 180 mm of water. The WBC count is 60/mm^3, 98% of which are mononuclear cells (mostly lymphocytes), the protein is 100 mg/dL, glucose is 40 mg/dL (concomitant blood glucose is 80 mg/dL). Examination of Gram-stained and India ink-stained CSF sediment preparations revealed no organism. The patient denied having taken any type of antibiotics since he felt sick. Which one of the following interventions is LEAST indicated in this patient?

(A) Administer a tuberculin skin test
(B) Collect blood for culture
(C) Send blood and CSF for *Mycobacterial* cultures
(D) Send CSF for a cryptococcal latex agglutination test
(E) Start chloramphenicol and high-dose ampicillin therapy immediately

75. Antibacterial agents will NOT be effective against which one of these venereal diseases?

(A) Chancroid
(B) Granuloma inguinale
(C) Lymphogranuloma venereum
(D) Molluscum contagiosum
(E) Syphilis

ANSWER KEY

1. B	16. D	31. B	46. B	61. D
2. A	17. E	32. A	47. E	62. C
3. C	18. E	33. E	48. B	63. E
4. B	19. C	34. B	49. B	64. B
5. A	20. E	35. D	50. C	65. A
6. B	21. B	36. D	51. C	66. B
7. A	22. B	37. B	52. E	67. C
8. C	23. D	38. C	53. E	68. B
9. B	24. C	39. D	54. A	69. E
10. C	25. E	40. E	55. B	70. E
11. C	26. C	41. E	56. B	71. E
12. C	27. B	42. B	57. B	72. A
13. C	28. C	43. E	58. E	73. D
14. C	29. B	44. D	59. A	74. E
15. B	30. E	45. D	60. A	75. D

ANSWERS AND EXPLANATIONS

Note: Page numbers designated as "IMI 4th Ed" refer to *Introduction to Medical Immunology,* 4th ed., New York/Basel, Marcel Dekker, 1998. Page numbers designated as "NMS M&ID 3rd Ed" refer to *NMS Microbiology and Infectious Diseases,* 3rd ed. Baltimore, Williams & Wilkins, 1997. Page numbers indicated as "PAInfDis 4th Ed" refer to Reese RE, Betts RF, eds., *Practical Approach to Infectious Diseases,* 4th ed., Boston, Little, Brown & Co., 1996.

1. The answer is B. This child has a rash typical of scarlet fever, and the tongue, described as "strawberry tongue," is also characteristically seen in scarlet fever. The causative agent is a lysogenized *Streptococcus pyogenes,* which carries a phage coding for pyrogenic (erythrogenic) toxin C. There are examples of virulence factors encoded by bacterial chromosomes, plasmids, and transposons, and it is possible that a generalized transducing phage could carry a virulence factor gene, but none of those mechanisms apply to the toxins responsible for scarlet fever. (NMS M&ID 3rd Ed., p. 105–8)

2. The answer is A. The pyrogenic toxins can cause fever by two mechanisms: a direct effect on the hypothalamus and indirectly, by promoting the release of pro-inflammatory cytokines (IL-1, TNFα, and others) from activated monocytes and T lymphocytes. Endotoxin (lipopolysaccharides) can also induce the release of pro-inflammatory cytokines, but streptococci are gram-positive organisms. M protein plays an important role as a major virulence factor, but it does not induce fever, either directly or indirectly. (NMS M&ID 3rd Ed., p. 107–8; IMI 4th Ed., p. 251–2)

3. The answer is C. With the notable exception of *Streptococcus pneumoniae,* streptococci are exquisitely sensitive to penicillin G. Erythromycin can be used when the patient is allergic to penicillin. Cephalosporins and vancomycin are not indicated, on the basis of cost, toxicity, or both. Obviously, supportive therapy is not sufficient. (NMS M&ID 3rd Ed., p. 105–12)

4. The answer is B. The clinical picture is one of neonatal bacterial meningitis, which in the majority of cases is caused by *E. coli* (a gram-negative rod), Group B *Streptococcus* (a gram-positive coccus), or *Listeria monocytogene*s (a gram-positive rod). The figure depicts a gram-positive coccus growing in chains, which would rank Group B streptococcus as the most likely candidate. The remaining listed characteristics (i.e., β-hemolysis, resistance to bacitracin, and positivity in the CAMP test) support the identification of the organism as Group B streptococcus. (NMS M&ID, 3rd Ed., p. 107–10, 430–4) The CAMP test, named for Christie, Atkins, and

Munch-Peterson, is a test in which *Staphylococcus* and *Streptococcus* are streaked perpendicularly in an agar plate, without allowing the 2 streaks to touch. If the streaked *Streptococcus* belongs to Group B, it releases a soluble factor (CAMP factor) that enhances the activity of the staphylococcal β-lysin, so in the area where the 2 streaks are in closer proximity, an enhancement of β-hemolysis can be seen, which will not be seen if the *Streptococcus* belongs to some other group. (NMS M&ID, 3rd Ed., p. 429–36)

5. The answer is A. All Group A and Group B streptococci are susceptible to penicillin, and resistance has never been reported. In contrast, *Streptococcus pneumoniae,* enterococci, and *Staphylococcus aureus* have acquired penicillin resistance, and vancomycin is often preferred for empiric therapy while antibiotic susceptibility tests are being run. Erythromycin can be used to treat streptococcal infections in patients allergic to penicillin, but is not the antibiotic of choice in normal conditions. (NMS M&ID 3rd Ed., p. 107–12)

6. The answer is B. The organism in the Gram stain is easily identifiable as extracellular and gram-positive. In the lower third of the picture, at the center, some isolated cocci can be distinguished, and the longer forms are likely to be duplets. Most likely the organism is *Streptococcus pneumoniae* and of the listed tests, the one that would certainly allow its identification would be the bile solubility test. Bacitracin susceptibility is used to differentiate *Streptococcus pyogenes* from other streptococci; hemolysis pattern is useful for differentiating streptococci other than *S. pneumoniae;* indole fermentation is used to differentiate *E. coli* from other coliforms; oxidase positivity is characteristic of *Neisseria, Pseudomonas,* and *Vibrio cholerae.* (NMS M&ID 3rd Ed., p. 110–12)

7. The answer is A. It is safer to assume that this could be a penicillin-resistant strain and start treatment with a third-generation cephalosporin, such as ceftriaxone, which is resistant to most penicillinases. Depending on the prevalence of cephalosporin-resistant strains in the locale where the patient fell ill, vancomycin may be preferred to start empiric therapy. Chloramphenicol and gentamicin do not offer any advantage over a third-generation cephalosporin and are considerably more toxic. (NMS M&ID 3rd Ed., p. 112)

8. The answer is C. The clinical vignette is suggestive of chronic granulomatous disease. Catalase-positive (catalase⁺) aerobic bacteria and fungi such as *Aspergillus* typically cause the infections that affect these patients. The figure shows gram-positive cocci that exist as singles or aggregates of different sizes, some of which resemble grape clusters—suggestive of staphylococci, which are catalase⁺ organisms. The molecular defect of the disease is, in most cases, a lack or abnormality of one of the two polypeptide proteins that forms cytochrome B. This abnormality interferes with the assembly of a functional nicotinamide adenine dinucleotide phosphate (NADPH) oxidase on the phagosome membrane, and this, in turn, results in inability to kill ingested organisms. Antibody or complement deficiencies can also be associated with increased frequency of bacterial infections, but fungi are not frequently involved. A severe lack of CD4+ cells is usually associated with severe combined immunodeficiency and a totally different clinical picture. Lack of phagosome formation, the basic abnormality in Chédiak-Higashi syndrome, is associated with striking morphological abnormalities, which should have been visible on the lymph node needle aspirate. (IMI 4th Ed., p.321–2, 329–31; NMS 3rd Ed., p. 346)

9. The answer is B. The previous answer points to chronic granulomatous disease. Cytochrome B is a cytochrome of the respiratory chain, a deficiency of which leads to chronic granulomatous disease. The other choices are enzymes that add phosphates to certain proteins (Bruton's tyrosine kinase), or help destroy cell walls (lysozyme); nitric synthetases are involved in the synthesis of nitric oxide, not affected in chronic granulomatous disease; and ZAP kinases initiate the intracellular signaling cascade in T cells. (IMI 4th Ed., p. 321–2)

10. The answer is C. There is no specific therapy for patients with chronic granulomatous disease. Prophylactic administration of sulfamethoxazole-trimethoprim seems to reduce the incidence of opportunistic bacterial infections. None of the other therapeutic interventions listed has been proven useful in these patients. (IMI 4th Ed., p. 329–31)

11. The answer is C. The administration of interferon-γ has been shown to reduce the incidence of opportunistic infections in patients with chronic granulomatous disease, particularly with the autosomal recessive form of the disease. Interferon-γ activates normal

macrophages, which show an increased respiratory burst, but the mechanism responsible for the beneficial effect in patients with chronic granulomatous disease is not known. Ascorbic acid is recommended in cases of another phagocytic defect, the Chédiak-Higashi syndrome. Granulocyte-macrophage colony-stimulating factor and the interleukins are not useful in this situation. (IMI 4th Ed., p. 321–3, 329–31).

12. The answer is C. The figure reproduces a very exuberant example of genital warts, most frequently caused by papilloma viruses of genotypes 6 and 11. Genotypes 16 and 18 are most frequently detected in cervical carcinoma tissues. Human herpesvirus 8 has been reported to be the cause of Kaposi's sarcoma. (NMS M&ID 3rd Ed., p. 285–6)

13. The answer is C. The figure illustrates a vesicular rash with dermatomal distribution, typical of shingles, caused by the varicella-zoster virus, which is one of the members of the herpes group. All human herpesviruses are enveloped, their nucleocapsid has icosahedral symmetry, and their genome is constituted by double-stranded DNA. (NMS M&ID 3rd Ed., p. 205–9)

14. The answer is C. The figure shows a single vesicular lesion in the finger and similar lesions are reported to be seen on the hard palate. This presentation is typical of hand-foot-and-mouth disease (without foot involvement, one of the areas may not be obviously involved), most frequently caused by Coxsackie A viruses, which are also a frequent cause of infantile diarrhea. Myocarditis and pleurodynia are also caused by a Coxsackie virus, most frequently type B. Cervical carcinoma and genital warts are caused by papillomaviruses. (NMS M&ID 3rd Ed., p. 296)

15. The answer is B. The clinical picture is suggestive of shingles and the finding of multinucleated giant cells on the base of a vesicle further reinforces that diagnosis. Varicella-zoster virus is relatively easy to grow and, as a rule, viral culture is the gold standard for diagnosis of a viral infection. Some of the other alternatives would be acceptable, except that they were aimed at the wrong viruses (Guarnieri inclusion bodies, located in the cytoplasm, are characteristic of poxviruses; HSV 1 and HSV 2 are not the cause of shingles). Finally, there is no good reason to order an HIV viral load to clarify the origin of a vesicular rash in a patient receiving chemotherapy for an inoperable tumor. (NMS M&ID 3rd Ed., p. 247–9, 279–80)

16. The answer is D. Most DNA viruses replicate in the nucleus, which is the most likely location of inclusion bodies. The exception is poxviruses, which replicate in the cytoplasm, and usually show intracytoplasmic inclusion bodies. B cell immortalization is usually caused by Epstein-Barr virus, lytic infections are characteristic of naked viruses (all viruses of the herpes group are enveloped), and the T antigens are encoded by polyomaviruses. (NMS M&ID 3rd Ed., p. 279–80)

17. The answer is E. The photograph shows a vesicular rash on the penis shaft, typical of genital herpes, which is caused by HSV, type 2. The recurrences of the rash are from reactivation of a latent infection in a regional sensory ganglion. The immune response is ineffective against integrated, latent viruses. This is the main mechanism of evasion for HSV 1 and HSV 2, which do not undergo antigenic variation. HSV may become resistant to antiviral agents, but not very frequently. (NMS M&ID 3rd Ed., p. 277–8)

18. The answer is E. The only effective measure to prevent sexual spread of the disease is the use of barrier contraceptives. Topical administration of famciclovir or treatment of the lesions with interferon-α are not effective to promote cure and do not guarantee future lack of transmission. Immunoprophylaxis is impossible because there is no effective vaccine. Prophylactic administration of acyclovir to the patient and his contacts for a long period of time would be expensive, hard to enforce, and may lead to the emergence of resistant strains. (NMS M&ID 3rd Ed., p. 279, 477–8)

19. The answer is C. Three acid-fast sporozoans can be involved in outbreaks of infectious diarrhea: *Cryptosporidium parvum, Cyclospora cayetanensis,* and *Isospora belli. I. belli* has not been associated with outbreaks of infectious diarrhea, and its oocysts are large and oval shaped, containing 2 spherical sporoblasts. The outbreaks of *C. cayetanensis* in the United States have been associated with ingestion of contaminated fruits or vegetables, an unlikely possibility in a large hospital when the affected patients range from the very young to the very old. *Cryptosporidium parvum,* in contrast, has been associated with some large outbreaks via contaminated water supply, which would appear considerably more likely in the scenario presented. All of these organisms tend to cause more severe disease in debilitated or immunocompromised patients. Amebiasis and giardiasis have not been reported as causes of waterborne outbreaks in the United States in recent memory. (NMS M&ID 3rd Ed., p. 387–8)

20. The answer is E. *Cryptosporidium parvum* is a common parasite of domestic livestock and its oocysts may contaminate the water supply from farm waste runoff. Contaminated vegetables or berries would be a likely vehicle for *Cyclospora cayetanensis.* Contaminated meat could be a vehicle for trichinosis (caused by *Trichinella*). (NMS M&ID 3rd Ed., p. 387–8)

21. The answer is B. A febrile immunocompromised patient with oral thrush and a perineal rash, neutropenia (200/mm^3) , receiving broad-spectrum antibiotics without apparent benefit, should be considered a very likely candidate to have systemic candidiasis. All the other listed fungi can be involved in opportunistic infections, but not systemic ones, and the relationship with neutropenia is stronger with *Candida albicans* than with any other fungus. (NMS M&ID 3rd Ed., p. 347–8, 357–9; IMI 4th Ed., 323–4, 505–6)

22. The answer is B. In this patient, the overriding question is whether he has developed systemic candidiasis, and the best way to evaluate this possibility is by requesting blood cultures in Sabouraud's agar, the medium of choice to grow most fungi. A KOH preparation of the material seen in the oral mucosal lesions could help to determine that the lesions were those of thrush, but would not add much information about the presence or absence of a systemic infection. Fecal cultures in MacConkey's and blood agars make little sense because this is not a case of bacterial gastroenteritis. Fecal cultures in Sabouraud's agar also make little sense, because *Candida albicans* is part of the intestinal normal flora. Serological tests for *C. albicans* do not give very good information about the nature of the infections (acute versus chronic, mucosal versus systemic). (NMS M&ID 3rd Ed., p. 339–40, 347–8)

23. The answer is D. The clinical picture of a recurrent febrile disease associated with hemolytic anemia (increased conjugated and total bilirubin, decreased haptoglobin, and traces of hemoglobin in the urine) and ring forms in the red cells is virtually diagnostic of malaria. The fact that the infected red cell is enlarged and contains granules (Schüffner's dots) allows identification of *Plasmodium vivax* as the cause of this patient's disease. *Plasmodium falciparum* is easily identified when banana-shaped gametocytes are visible in the peripheral blood. Infected cells show ring stages, but do not show Schüffner's dots. Of the other listed parasites, only *Babesia* could cause a similar clinical picture, but that is not a tropical or subtropical parasite, tends to infect splenectomized patients, and the infection is not as severe as malaria. (NMS M&ID 3rd Ed., p. 339–40).

24. The answer is C. The figure shows skin lesions that appear to be flat, poorly pigmented, and without apparent perilesional or intralesional inflammation. This is a typical presentation of tinea versicolor, caused by *Malassezia furfur*. The rash of Lyme disease (caused by *Borrelia burgdorferi*) is described as annular, more intense in the periphery, and is usually not as well circumscribed. The rashes of measles and streptococcal scarlet fever are not hypopigmented, and very different in aspect. The lesions of tuberculoid leprosy (caused by *Mycobacterium leprae*) may be hypopigmented, but usually have a raised, erythematous edge, which cannot be seen in this patient. (NMS M&ID 3rd Ed., p. 108, 173, 181–2, 344, 491)

25. The answer is E. This girl presents with fever and a vesicular rash which starts in the trunk and spreads to the face, highly suggestive of chickenpox. The lesions in the picture are of different sizes, which is also typical of chickenpox, caused by the varicella-zoster virus. The lesions caused by HSV type 1 are usually perioral and would not start in the trunk. The rash associated with measles is maculopapular and starts in the face, spreading to the trunk and extremities. Coxsackie A virus infections may be associated with a vesicular rash, are usually scanty, and do not affect the trunk. The lesions of bacterial impetigo (which can be caused by *Streptococcus pyogenes*) may be vesicular, but the contents are purulent, tend to break, ooze, form crusts, and remain localized. (NMS M&ID 3rd Ed., p. 103, 491–6)

26. The answer is C. The clinical case is suggestive of serum sickness with joint and kidney involvement and cutaneous vasculitis. Both hepatitis B and hepatitis C can present with these type of symptoms, from the deposition of soluble immune complexes. One of the easier techniques for detecting circulating immune complexes is cold precipitation of mixed cryoglobulins, generally constituted by viral antigens, IgM antibodies, and IgM rheumatoid factors. This is not a very sensitive assay, but it is very specific for soluble immune complexes. Other tests may or may not be positive and in a patient with hepatitis C, depending on the degree of liver involvement (high bilirubin) or of viral involvement secondary to deposition of immune complexes (casts, proteinuria). Positive rheumatoid factor is too unspecific, and most often associated with rheumatoid arthritis.(NMS M&ID 3rd Ed., p. 326; IMI 4th Ed., 484–7)

27. The answer is B. To this day there has been no effective therapy developed for treating chronic hepatitis infections. But in the case of hepatitis C virus, being a (+)RNA virus, a protease inhibitor that would effectively prevent the processing of viral polyproteins could be an effective therapy. Actually, therapeutic trials with protease inhibitors are being conducted. (NMS M&ID 3rd Ed., p. 238, 330)

28. The answer is C. HDV is a defective virus that depends on HBV for its replication. Therefore, it either co-

infects with HBV or superinfects an HBV-positive individual. Intravenous drug abusers are at special risk for HDV superinfection that can result in a severe form of hepatitis, with greater mortality than when HBV is exclusively involved. (NMS M&ID 3rd Ed., p. 330–1)

29. The answer is B. The patient has a history of jaundice followed by a serum sickness-like syndrome, with joint pains and generalized skin lesions that slowly subsided. This is highly suggestive of hepatitis B, and it becomes particularly important to check whether this patient is a carrier because of the possibility of transmission to the newborn. Actually, testing for HB_sAg is recommended as part of routine prenatal care. HIV screening is also recommended, but not because of a specific clinical history. Malaria is an unlikely choice because the clinical findings are not suggestive and there is no mention of a history of travel to areas of high prevalence. IgM serologies would not help to clarify the etiology of a disease that has followed a 3-year course. (NMS M&ID 3rd Ed., p. 481)

30. The answer is E. The symptoms—indurated and painless penile ulceration—are suggestive of primary syphilis. Because *Treponema pallidum* cannot be cultured or visualized by conventional staining, the usual approach is to order one of the screening serological tests, such as the Venereal Disease Research Laboratory (VDRL) test. The VDRL, being a flocculation test, is well suited for the purpose because it will detect IgM antibodies very early in the disease. *Treponema*-specific tests such as the microhemagglutination *Treponema pallidum* test (MHA-TP) are reserved as confirmatory tests for cases where there may be reason to question the result of the screening test. (NMS M&ID 3rd Ed., p. 178, 475)

31. The answer is B. The clinical picture is suggestive of pelvic inflammatory disease (PID), which can develop as a complication of gonococcal infection or of nongonococcal urethritis. However, in many cases the infection of the adnexa and surrounding peritoneum may involve both *Neisseria gonorrhoeae* and *Chlamydia trachomatis,* and even some other bacteria. The treatment of PID is medical, and is initiated empirically, taking into consideration the etiologic possibilities. It should include at least one third-generation cephalosporin effective against *N. gonorrhoeae* and many other gram-negative organisms, and doxycycline, to cover *C. trachomatis.* Usually treatment will be started as soon as the diagnosis is suspected, and the results of bacteriological cultures will be used to determine possible adjustments to the treatment. The possibility of septic shock is not very likely, at least when *N. gonorrhoeae* and *C. trachomatis* are the only organisms involved, as neither one is likely to cause septic shock. Toxic-shock secreting *Staphylococcus aureus* could obviously cause shock, by releasing toxic shock syndrome toxin-1, a potent superantigen. However, *S. aureus* is not usually involved as an agent of PID. (NMS M&ID 3rd Ed., p. 130–2, 196–7, 478)

32. The answer is A. Among the listed conditions, infertility is the most likely complication resulting from pelvic inflammatory disease (PID). The inflammatory process affecting the fallopian tubes and surrounding tissues may result in scarring and stricture, leading to infertility. The perihepatitis (Fitz-Hugh and Curtis syndrome) that may develop in patients with PID does not usually leave sequelae. (NMS M&ID 3rd Ed., p. 478)

33. The answer is E. On a global scale, HIV infection is more prevalent among populations with low socioeconomic status. Age, gender, race, and sexual preference differences do exist in different areas of the world, but none of those factors has as strong a correlation with the incidence of AIDS on the global scale as low socioeconomic status. (NMS M&ID 3rd Ed., p. 503)

34. The answer is B. The introduction of the *Haemophilus influenzae* type B vaccine (HiB) conjugate vaccine in the 1990s has been followed by a marked decrease in the frequency of severe infections caused by *H. influenzae,* exceeding the projections relative to the percentage of the population that has been immunized. (NMS M&ID 3rd Ed., p. 135, 430)

35. The answer is D. The presentation of fever (39°C), malaise, anorexia, and flank pain is suggestive of pyelonephritis. This diagnosis is supported by the history of recent bladder catheterization (which most likely was the source of infection by an opportunistic agent) and by the finding of pus cells and casts in the urine. Cystitis is usually not associated with fever and flank pain or with casts in the urinary sediment. The typical presentation of an acute glomerulonephritis includes hematuria, edema, and hypertension. The possibility of an associated bacteremia can only be ruled out by blood cultures, but the patient had a clinical picture suggestive of pyelonephritis but not of bacteremia. Urethritis is not clinically seen in women. (NMS M&ID 3rd Ed., p. 449–52)

36. The answer is D. The description of an oxidase-positive, gram-negative rod that released a green diffusible pigment would fit with *Pseudomonas aeruginosa* and not with any other of the listed bacteria. *Pseudomonas* is also a likely organism to be introduced with a urethral catheter, given its ubiquitous nature and, resistance to disinfectants.(NMS M&ID 3rd Ed., p. 160–2)

37. The answer is B. In investigating a possible hepatitis, the most frequent causes should always be kept in mind (ruling out Lyme disease, malaria, relapsing fever, as highly unlikely). In this patient, serologies for hepatitis A and B were negative. A veterinarian, on the other hand, is exposed to occupational diseases, such as leptospirosis, which can be contracted from the urine of infected dogs. The symptoms include headaches, myalgia, nausea, vomiting. In severe cases the patients develop disseminated endothelial damage, which leads to multiple organ involvement including the liver (hepatic inflammation and jaundice) and the kidney (impairment of tubular function). (NMS M&ID 3rd Ed., p. 183–4)

38. The answer is C. The agent of leptospirosis, *Leptospira interrogans,* is eliminated in the urine of infected dogs. Animal handlers, veterinarians, and so forth are at risk of exposure to this agent. (NMS M&ID 3rd Ed., p. 183–4).

39. The answer is D. Acute bronchopneumonia in young children is often of viral origin, the most frequent offender being the respiratory syncytial virus. The finding of large multinucleated cellular clumps (syncytia) in the nasopharyngeal swab further reinforces this diagnostic impression, which can be confirmed or ruled out with a rapid enzyme immunoassay that can be performed in a few minutes. In contrast, both bacterial and viral cultures will take at least 24 hours. The Gram stain and acid-fast stains are relatively fast, but bacteria are not likely to be involved. A cold agglutinin titer can be obtained in a few hours, but *Mycoplasma* is not likely to be involved either. (NMS M&ID 3rd Ed., p. 309, 313)

40. The answer is E. All of the listed organisms can cause pneumonia, but *Pneumocystis carinii* is the most likely one to be involved in an HIV-positive patient, particularly when the patient presents with hypoxemia (suggested by cyanosis), a very common feature in *P. carinii* pneumonia, and the radiograph shows bilateral interstitial infiltrates. *Chlamydia,* CMV, and HSV can also cause interstitial pneumonia, but are considerably less frequently involved. (NMS M&ID 3rd Ed., p. 425–26, 509)

41. The answer is E. Trimethoprim-sulfamethoxazole is the therapy of choice for *Pneumocystis carinii* pneumonia. Pentamidine and dapsone are unlisted alternatives, only indicated when the patient cannot tolerate or fails to respond to trimethoprim–sulfamethoxazole. All other listed agents are not effective against *P. carinii.* (NMS M&ID 3rd Ed., p. 388, 425–6, 513)

42. The answer is B. There is no question about the need to start antiretroviral therapy as soon as possible after diagnosis. Because of possible teratogenic effects (not reported), therapy is withheld until 14 weeks of gestation. Zidovudine administered during pregnancy has been proven to significantly reduce the risk of maternofetal transmission. As for the decision about whether to start high-activity antiretroviral therapy with the association of three antiretroviral drugs, the benefit of reducing the viral load to undetectable levels seems to outweigh the possible risk of teratogenic effects, not very likely after week 14. (NMS M&ID 3rd Ed., p. 511–2)

43. The answer is E. The risk of maternofetal transmission varies in different geographic areas. In the United States, it is estimated to be around 25%–30% without treatment, and to be reduced to about 8% with proper treatment, which includes administering zidovudine to the mother during pregnancy and during birth, and postpartum administration to the child, who should continue to receive zidovudine during the first 6 months of life. (NMS M&ID 3rd Ed., p. 511)

44. The answer is D. Vertical transmission can occur during pregnancy, at birth, and through breast feeding. Most cases of maternofetal transmission of HIV occur perinatally, that is, close to the time of birth, either during birth because of exposure to maternal blood and secretions infected with the virus, or during the later stages of uterine development, from transplacental transmission of the virus. Third in frequency is transmission from breast feeding. (PAInfDis, 4th Ed., p. 88–9)

45. The answer is D. The presentation is strongly suggestive of staphylococcal toxic shock syndrome, which is caused by *Staphylococcus aureus* strains able to release the toxic shock syndrome toxin-1 (TSST-1). This toxin is a "superantigen" able to cross-link MHC-II molecules on macrophages and other antigen-presenting cells with the T cell receptors of specific structural families shared by a large proportion of T cells. The mutual activation of T cells and macrophages promoted by the superantigen-mediated interaction results in the release of large amounts of pro-inflammatory cytokines (IL-1, TNFα, and others), which cause most of the symptoms of toxic shock. Dissolution of red cell membranes and hemolysis are caused by *Clostridium perfringens* α toxin; epidermolysis is classically caused by a related staphylococcal exotoxin, know as exfoliatin. (NMS M&ID 3rd Ed., p. 69, 102, 104, 118, 415; IMI 4th Ed., 251–2)

46. The answer is B. Opportunistic infections are defined as those caused by bacteria that are members of the normal flora or commonly found in the environment and that may cause severe systemic infection. *Brucella, Giardia, H. pylori,* and *Mycobacterium tuberculosis* are true

pathogenic organisms and the listed associations have to do with professional exposure or with genetic predisposition. In contrast, *E. coli* bacteremia in an immunocompromised patient is a very good example of opportunistic infection; as a rule, the *E. coli* is not acquired from exogenous sources but rather from the individual's endogenous flora. In normal circumstances bacteria do reach the circulation but are quickly eliminated. In immunocompromised patients the bacteria that reach the circulation have a better chance to multiply and cause bacteremia. (NMS M&ID 3rd Ed., p. 141–2, 159, 410–1)

47. The answer is E. Viral encephalitis is a disease with considerable morbidity and mortality, particularly when HSV is involved. In this patient the possible involvement of arboviruses looks unlikely (no history of exposure to vector, no outbreak in the community), leaving as more likely possibilities HSV or one of the enteroviruses. The inconclusive result of the frontal lobe biopsy does not allow herpes simplex to be ruled out, and therefore, acyclovir therapy should be initiated immediately, without excluding some of the other listed interventions. (NMS M&ID 3rd Ed., p. 278–9, 439)

48. The answer is B. When a migrant worker presents with a febrile disease, it is important to consider diseases that may not be common in the United States but are common in other parts of the Western hemisphere. In this case the presentation could be compatible with malaria and perhaps with other parasitic diseases. These possibilities were not supported by the results of blood examinations and of search for eggs and parasites in fecal material. On the other hand, there is a history of occupational exposure to sheep and the results of the hemogram suggest either a viral infection or infection by an intracellular bacteria (in both cases, cell-mediated immunity is the primary mechanism of defense once the infection is established). With these elements, and considering that the patient is suffering from recurrent fever, brucellosis should be considered as a very likely possibility. The clinical picture of salmonellosis or trypanosomiasis, on the other hand, is totally different. (NMS M&ID 3rd Ed., p. 162–4; IMI 4th Ed., 246–7)

49. The answer is B. The transmission of brucellosis involves either direct contact with contaminated animal products by meat handlers and veterinarians, or ingestion of contaminated goat and cheese milk or cheese. However, the contamination of food arises from the animal infection, not from an infected food handler. (NMS M&ID 3rd Ed., p. 162–3)

50. The answer is C. The CD4 count was the first surrogate marker used to evaluate the effects of antiretroviral therapy, but it has been replaced in the last 2 years by assays of the viral load, which basically measure the number of copies of viral RNA in circulation, using a variety of techniques to amplify the nucleic acid and to detect it with an adequate probe. There is considerable interest in determining the residual infected cell population after therapy has induced disappearance of the circulating virus, and the number of infected cells in lymph nodes could be such a parameter, but practical obstacles may prevent its use in clinical practice. Viral culture and the assay of viral antigens in circulation have been tried but abandoned because of technical problems, which result in unreliable data. (IMI 4th Ed., p. 609)

51. The answer is C. Currently, only one immunization is recommended at the time of birth—the hepatitis B vaccine. The next set of immunizations, given at 2 months of age, includes a second dose of the hepatitis B vaccine, as well as the first doses of diphtheria-tetanus-acellular pertussis (DTaP), polio vaccine, and conjugated *Haemophilus influenzae* vaccine (HiB). The first dose of measles-mumps-rubella (MMR) is given at 1 year of age. (NMS M&ID 3rd Ed., p. 86)

52. The answer is E. The clinical picture and laboratory data strongly suggest that this neonate has a bacterial infection. Blood cultures should be obtained, and a diagnosis of meningitis should be explored. After evaluating clinically, or through a computed tomography scan, the possible presence of increased intracranial pressure, CSF should be obtained for Gram stain, cell count, and cultures. Empiric antibiotherapy should be initiated as soon as samples for culture were collected, covering the bacteria most likely to infect a neonate—*E. coli,* group B *Streptococcus,* and *Listeria monocytogenes.* Enteroviral cultures of the CSF do not appear to have the same priority, because the leukocytosis with predominance of neutrophils and bands strongly suggests that the infection is bacterial, and the treatment of this child cannot be postponed until the results of these cultures become available. (NMS M&ID 3rd Ed., p. 429–33)

53. The answer is E. The main clue to this case is the elevated titers of antimeasles hemagglutinin antibody, which are characteristic of subacute sclerosing panencephalitis, caused by persistent infection of the central nervous system by measles virus. The findings on the MRI are also suggestive. Confirmation of the diagnosis requires brain biopsy, but none of the other diseases listed would be associated with the described clinical and laboratory findings. (NMS M&ID 3rd Ed., p. 441–7).

54. The answer is A. The clinical symptoms are suggestive of cholera and the flight originated in Lima, Peru, the epicenter of a major cholera epidemic. Raw vegetables, such as those in a garden salad, are a very

likely vehicle for *Vibrio cholerae.* Shrimp could be a second possibility, but shrimp cocktail is prepared with boiled shrimp, which should be safe. (NMS M&ID 3rd Ed., p. 151–4)

55. The answer is B. The most important measure in all secretory diarrheas, such as cholera, is to administer fluids and electrolytes to avoid dehydration. The diagnosis is clinical and does not require confirmation, except for epidemiological purposes. Antimicrobial therapy is not indicated; this type of diarrhea is self-limiting. Antidiarrheal medications are totally ineffective and should not be used, in any event, because diarrhea is an effective defense mechanism, promoting elimination of the infecting organism. (NMS M&ID 3rd Ed., p. 154, 456–9)

56. The answer is B. This patient has an invasive type of diarrhea, as indicated by the finding of mucus, inflammatory cells, and erythrocytes in the feces. Viral diarrheas are of the secretory type and self-limiting, and investigating a viral cause for this patient's diarrhea is totally unwarranted. All other choices could correspond to invasive diarrheas, including the enteroinvasive and enterohemorrhagic strains of *E. coli.* (NMS M&ID 3rd Ed., p. 143–51, 456–62)

57. The answer is B. The clinical case is strongly suggestive of infectious mononucleosis, and a positive test for heterophile hemagglutinins (the monospot test) is confirmatory, although not totally specific. The responsible agent is Epstein-Barr virus in the vast majority of cases. CMV can cause a mononucleosis-like disease, but usually in association with organ transplantation or blood transfusions. The three listed bacteria can cause sore throat but not the other symptoms and findings seen in this patient, particularly generalized lymphadenopathy, hepatosplenomegaly, and heterophile hemagglutinins. (NMS M&ID 3rd Ed., p. 280–2)

58. The answer is E. Although Epstein-Barr virus is a member of the herpes group, it is not susceptible to the antiviral agents used for treating infections caused by HSV and CMV. Therefore, the treatment is exclusively symptomatic. (NMS M&ID 3rd Ed., p. 277–82)

59. The answer is A. The clinical picture is suggestive of amebiasis, which evolved from predominantly intestinal to extraintestinal, with formation of a liver abscess (the most frequent extraintestinal manifestation of amebiasis). *Fasciola hepatica* causes blockage of the biliary ducts, but is not associated with diarrhea or intrahepatic lesions. *Salmonella enteritidis* and *Shigella sonnei* usually cause acute diarrhea that is self-limiting and the infection does not spread to the liver. *Schistosoma mansoni* can involve both the intestine and the liver, but does not cause the formation of liver abscesses. (NMS M&ID 3rd Ed., p. 371–2)

60. The answer is A. The best characterized virulence factor of *Entamoeba histolytica* is a cysteine protease that is believed to digest the extracellular matrix, allowing the parasite to invade a variety of tissues. The other listed virulence factors are released by a variety of bacteria, such as *Shigella* (intercellular spread protein), *Salmonella* (invasins), *E. coli* O157:H7 (Shiga-like toxin), and *H. pylori* (vacuolating cytotoxin). (NMS M&ID 3rd Ed., p. 371–2)

61. The answer is D. The most cost-effective method for preventing tetanus is, without question, proper immunization. Cleaning and débriding a wound and administering antibiotics immediately after the injury are routine procedures that may prevent an anaerobe from growing in the wound, and the remaining interventions may be part of the treatment of a tetanus-prone wound in a nonimmunized patient. None of those measures compares in efficiency to proper immunization, and their cost will always be higher because of the need to combine a variety of interventions. (NMS M&ID 3rd Ed., p. 121–3)

62. The answer is C. All of the diseases listed are transmitted by insect vectors, but only ehrlichiosis is transmitted by ticks. Bartonellosis and leishmaniasis are transmitted by flies, dengue by mosquitoes, and typhus by lice, fleas, or mites. (NMS M&ID 3rd Ed., p. 198–202)

63. The answer is E. All of the diseases listed are degenerative diseases of the brain of proven or hypothetical infectious etiology. Progressive spastic paraparesis is caused by HTLV-1, a retrovirus also associated with T cell leukemia. Bovine spongiform encephalopathy, Creutzfeldt-Jakob disease, and Kuru are diseases caused by prions; progressive multifocal encephalopathy is caused by the JC virus, which is a DNA virus. (NMS M&ID 3rd Ed., p. 441–7)

64. The answer is B. *Campylobacter jejuni* infection has been shown to be associated with the Guillain-Barré syndrome. This organism apparently induces an immune response in which antibodies directed to the bacterial endotoxin oligosaccharides cross-react with neuron gangliosides and cause an acute inflammatory demyelinating polyradiculopathy. Some viral diseases (influenza in particular) have also been reported to be associated with the Guillain-Barré syndrome but the actual molecular mechanism is not as well-characterized as in the case of *C. jejuni*. (NMS M&ID 3rd Ed., p. 155–6, 307)

65. The answer is A. The presentation is typical of chickenpox: young infant with fever and a maculovesic-

ular rash that predominates in the trunk, with lesions in different stages of evolution. The finding of vesicular lesions in the oral cavity is frequent, seen in nearly 50% of the children. Herpangina presents with vesicular lesions on the soft palate but lacks the skin rash. Measles and roseola have maculopapular rashes and the rash of scarlet fever is described as fine and papular, compared to sandpaper. (NMS M&ID 3rd Ed., p. 108, 491–2, 494–5)

66. The answer is B. In the context of an outbreak of jaundice on a day care center, hepatitis A would be a most likely possibility, certainly more likely than any of the other listed possibilities. Reye's syndrome emerging in a child with an acute viral disease after administration of aspirin can be associated with liver damage, but in this child the dose of aspirin appears to have been given after all the symptoms had emerged, not before. (NMS M&ID 3rd Ed., p. 307, 482–3)

67. The answer is C. In the vast majority of cases, hepatitis A is followed by complete recovery. If the diagnosis had been Reye's syndrome, progression to coma and risk of death would be a definite possibility. (NMS M&ID 3rd Ed., p. 307, 323–4)

68. The answer is B. Esophageal candidiasis is not seen in patients other than those who are HIV-positive, and is a marker of severe immunodepression. Thus, a patient with esophageal candidiasis fulfills the diagnostic criteria for AIDS. Recurrent vaginal candidiasis in females is a very strong indicator of AIDS, but does not have the same diagnostic weight, because recurrent candidiasis may also be seen in HIV-negative patients. Cryptococcal meningitis, pulmonary histoplasmosis, and *Salmonella* bacteremia are frequently seen in HIV-positive patients, but are also seen in patients without HIV infection, and as such, are not considered pathognomonic for AIDS. (NMS M&ID 3rd Ed., p. 510)

69. The answer is E. Infectious agents are believed to cause or at least to play a co-carcinogenic role in all the listed infections: HTLV-I causes adult T cell leukemia, *Schistosoma haematobium* is believed to cause bladder carcinoma, Epstein-Barr virus is associated with Burkitt's lymphoma, papilloma viruses are the apparent cause of cervical carcinoma, and HBV causes hepatoma. Of all these diseases, only hepatitis B can be effectively prevented by immunization. Obviously, if hepatitis B is effectively prevented, so will hepatoma. (NMS M&ID 3rd Ed., p. 251–60, 324–7, 402–3)

70. The answer is E. All of the infectious agents listed can cause congenital infections, although some do so more frequently than others. The combination of microcephaly, cerebral calcifications, and chorioretinitis is highly suggestive of congenital toxoplasmosis. Herpes simplex is transmitted transplacentally only in exceptional cases; most frequently it is transmitted perinatally, and presents with a vesicular rash. When the infection is acquired transplacentally, microcephaly and organomegaly are the most frequent clinical signs. Congenital rubella is rarely seen because of vaccination; the most typical symptoms include low birth weight, thrombocytopenia, organomegaly, microcephaly, cataracts, cardiac lesions, and deafness. Congenital syphilis affects mostly the bone and cartilage, leading to morphological abnormalities such as skeletal and craniofacial alterations including notched teeth, often associated with interstitial keratitis, deafness, hepatosplenomegaly. (NMS M&ID 3rd Ed., p. 177, 278–9, 302, 385)

71. The answer is E. *Campylobacter jejuni, E. coli* O157:H7, and *Giardia lamblia* may infect infants and young children, but none approaches rotavirus in morbidity among the very young. Rotavirus infection is associated with significant mortality when affecting very young infants. A vaccine against this virus has recently received Food and Drug Administration (FDA) approval. Norwalk virus typically occurs in adults and school-age children, and as such is not a cause of infantile morbidity. (NMS M&ID 3rd Ed., p. 460–1)

72. The answer is A. The clinical signs and symptoms suggest anaerobic pneumonia (dullness to percussion and absent breath sounds over the right posterior mid-lung field; fetid odor on his breath). The source of anaerobes in this situation is the gingivosulcal flora, rich in anaerobes. Aspiration of anaerobes from the stomach and intestine is only possible when the pH of the stomach is so abnormally high that it allows bacterial colonization or when intestinal contents reflux into the stomach, both very rare conditions that are unlikely to occur in a young college student. Translocation of intestinal bacteria usually happens mainly in situations of splanchnic ischemia, which are not likely to exist in this patient. Depressed ventilatory function could play a role, but not the main one. Immunodeficiency secondary to alcoholism is usually a consequence of chronic alcohol

abuse, and there is no clue about whether this patient is an alcoholic or just an immature juvenile involved in an episode of binge drinking. (NMS M&ID 3rd Ed., p. 98, 468–9; IMI 4th Ed., 603)

73. The answer is D. Most anaerobes are very sensitive to Penicillin G. *Bacteroides* species can be resistant to penicillin, but is not one of the organisms that is usually part of the normal anaerobic flora of the mouth. Therefore, penicillin G in high doses would be a good choice to start treatment, and other antibiotics should be reserved for cases that do not respond to penicillin. (NMS M&ID 3rd Ed., 470–71; PAInfDis, 4th Ed., p. 277–8)

74. The answer is E. The patient presents with symptoms that suggest meningitis, and a CSF examination reveals mild leukocytosis with lymphocyte predominance, elevated protein, and a sugar concentration on the lower end of normal. These findings are not compatible with a bacterial meningitis caused by pyogenic bacteria. Therefore, empiric therapy with chloramphenicol and ampicillin does not appear warranted, particularly because of the risk of serious side effects associated with administering chloramphenicol. Tuberculous meningitis could present with the symptoms and laboratory findings described in this patient. Thus, a tuberculin test and collecting blood and CSF for culture would appear indicated. Because negative findings never rule out a possibility, blood cultures should be ordered to further investigate possible bacteria, which could be the source of the meningeal infection, and testing for fungal antigens could be ordered, because those tests are more sensitive than the India ink test. (NMS M&ID 3rd Ed., p. 429–34).

75. The answer is D. Molluscum contagiosum is caused by a poxvirus of the *Leporipoxvirus* genus, and treatment with antibacterial drugs will obviously be ineffective. All the other choices are bacterial sexually transmitted diseases: chancroid is caused by *Haemophilus ducreyi,* granuloma inguinale by *Calymmatobacterium granulomatis,* lymphogranuloma venereum by *Chlamydia trachomatis,* and syphilis by *Treponema pallidum.* (NMS M&ID 3rd Ed., p. 291, 473–6)

Appendix: Normal Values

1. Serum immunoglobulins (mg/dL)

	IgG	IgA	IgM
Newborn	645–1244	0–11	5–30
One year	279–1533	16–98	22–147
Three to five years	569–1597	55–152	22–100
Adult	569–1919	61–330	47–147
IgE (Adult Level):	6–780 ng/dL		

2. Serum C3: 80–180 mg/dL

3. Carcinoembryonic antigen (CEA): Less than 2.5 ng/dL

4. Serum creatinine: 0.5–1.4 mg/dL

5. Hematologic values

Hemoglobin	Males	13.3–16.0 gm/dL
	Females	11.7–15.7 gm/dL
Erythrocytes	Males	4.4–5.9 million/μL
	Females	3.8–5.2 million/μL
WBC	3500–11,000/μL	
Differential	Neutrophils	55%–66%
	Lymphocytes	25%–33%
	Monocytes	3%–10%
	Eosinophils	1%–3%
	Basophils	0%–1%
Sedimentation rate	Males	0–5 mm in 1 hour
	Females	0–15 mm in 1 hour

6. Total serum protein: 6–8 g/dL

7. Total urinary protein: 10–150 mg/24 hours

8. Lymphocytes in peripheral blood

CD19	4%–20%	96–421 cells/μL
CD3	62%–85%	700–2500 cells/μL
CD2	70%–88%	840–2800 cells/μL
CD4	34%–59%	430–1600 cells/μL
CD8	16%–38%	280–1100 cells/μL

9. Mitogenic responses to incorporation of tritiated thymidine (^{3}H-Tdr)

	mean ± s.d
Phytohemagglutin (PHA)	15,000 ± 6,000 cpm
Concanavalin (ConA)	10,000 ± 2,000 cpm

10. Response to pokeweed mitogen (PWM)
    a. IgG: 2–5 mg/10^6 cells
    b. IgM: 3–12 mg/10^6 cells

11. C1q binding assay: ≤4 mEq Heat-aggregated IgG/mL

NMS Q&A: Microbiology, Immunology, and Infectious Diseases Answer Sheet

TEST 1: Immunology

1. A B C D E F G H I J
2. A B C D E F G H I J
3. A B C D E F G H I J
4. A B C D E F G H I J
5. A B C D E F G H I J
6. A B C D E F G H I J
7. A B C D E F G H I J
8. A B C D E F G H I J
9. A B C D E F G H I J
10. A B C D E F G H I J
11. A B C D E F G H I J
12. A B C D E F G H I J
13. A B C D E F G H I J
14. A B C D E F G H I J
15. A B C D E F G H I J
16. A B C D E F G H I J
17. A B C D E F G H I J
18. A B C D E F G H I J
19. A B C D E F G H I J
20. A B C D E F G H I J
21. A B C D E F G H I J
22. A B C D E F G H I J
23. A B C D E F G H I J
24. A B C D E F G H I J
25. A B C D E F G H I J
26. A B C D E F G H I J
27. A B C D E F G H I J
28. A B C D E F G H I J
29. A B C D E F G H I J
30. A B C D E F G H I J
31. A B C D E F G H I J
32. A B C D E F G H I J
33. A B C D E F G H I J
34. A B C D E F G H I J
35. A B C D E F G H I J
36. A B C D E F G H I J
37. A B C D E F G H I J
38. A B C D E F G H I J
39. A B C D E F G H I J
40. A B C D E F G H I J
41. A B C D E F G H I J
42. A B C D E F G H I J
43. A B C D E F G H I J
44. A B C D E F G H I J
45. A B C D E F G H I J
46. A B C D E F G H I J
47. A B C D E F G H I J
48. A B C D E F G H I J
49. A B C D E F G H I J
50. A B C D E F G H I J
51. A B C D E F G H I J
52. A B C D E F G H I J
53. A B C D E F G H I J
54. A B C D E F G H I J
55. A B C D E F G H I J
56. A B C D E F G H I J
57. A B C D E F G H I J
58. A B C D E F G H I J
59. A B C D E F G H I J
60. A B C D E F G H I J
61. A B C D E F G H I J
62. A B C D E F G H I J
63. A B C D E F G H I J
64. A B C D E F G H I J
65. A B C D E F G H I J
66. A B C D E F G H I J
67. A B C D E F G H I J
68. A B C D E F G H I J
69. A B C D E F G H I J
70. A B C D E F G H I J
71. A B C D E F G H I J
72. A B C D E F G H I J
73. A B C D E F G H I J
74. A B C D E F G H I J
75. A B C D E F G H I J
76. A B C D E F G H I J
77. A B C D E F G H I J
78. A B C D E F G H I J
79. A B C D E F G H I J
80. A B C D E F G H I J

TEST 2: Bacteriology

1. A B C D E F G H I J
2. A B C D E F G H I J
3. A B C D E F G H I J
4. A B C D E F G H I J
5. A B C D E F G H I J
6. A B C D E F G H I J
7. A B C D E F G H I J
8. A B C D E F G H I J
9. A B C D E F G H I J
10. A B C D E F G H I J
11. A B C D E F G H I J
12. A B C D E F G H I J
13. A B C D E F G H I J
14. A B C D E F G H I J
15. A B C D E F G H I J
16. A B C D E F G H I J
17. A B C D E F G H I J
18. A B C D E F G H I J
19. A B C D E F G H I J
20. A B C D E F G H I J
21. A B C D E F G H I J
22. A B C D E F G H I J
23. A B C D E F G H I J
24. A B C D E F G H I J
25. A B C D E F G H I J
26. A B C D E F G H I J
27. A B C D E F G H I J
28. A B C D E F G H I J
29. A B C D E F G H I J
30. A B C D E F G H I J
31. A B C D E F G H I J
32. A B C D E F G H I J
33. A B C D E F G H I J
34. A B C D E F G H I J
35. A B C D E F G H I J
36. A B C D E F G H I J
37. A B C D E F G H I J
38. A B C D E F G H I J
39. A B C D E F G H I J
40. A B C D E F G H I J
41. A B C D E F G H I J
42. A B C D E F G H I J
43. A B C D E F G H I J
44. A B C D E F G H I J
45. A B C D E F G H I J
46. A B C D E F G H I J
47. A B C D E F G H I J
48. A B C D E F G H I J
49. A B C D E F G H I J
50. A B C D E F G H I J
51. A B C D E F G H I J
52. A B C D E F G H I J
53. A B C D E F G H I J
54. A B C D E F G H I J
55. A B C D E F G H I J
56. A B C D E F G H I J
57. A B C D E F G H I J
58. A B C D E F G H I J
59. A B C D E F G H I J
60. A B C D E F G H I J
61. A B C D E F G H I J
62. A B C D E F G H I J
63. A B C D E F G H I J
64. A B C D E F G H I J
65. A B C D E F G H I J
66. A B C D E F G H I J
67. A B C D E F G H I J
68. A B C D E F G H I J
69. A B C D E F G H I J
70. A B C D E F G H I J
71. A B C D E F G H I J
72. A B C D E F G H I J
73. A B C D E F G H I J
74. A B C D E F G H I J
75. A B C D E F G H I J
76. A B C D E F G H I J
77. A B C D E F G H I J
78. A B C D E F G H I J
79. A B C D E F G H I J
80. A B C D E F G H I J
81. A B C D E F G H I J
82. A B C D E F G H I J
83. A B C D E F G H I J
84. A B C D E F G H I J
85. A B C D E F G H I J

TEST 3: Virology

1. A B C D E F G H I J
2. A B C D E F G H I J
3. A B C D E F G H I J
4. A B C D E F G H I J
5. A B C D E F G H I J
6. A B C D E F G H I J
7. A B C D E F G H I J
8. A B C D E F G H I J
9. A B C D E F G H I J
10. A B C D E F G H I J
11. A B C D E F G H I J
12. A B C D E F G H I J
13. A B C D E F G H I J
14. A B C D E F G H I J
15. A B C D E F G H I J
16. A B C D E F G H I J
17. A B C D E F G H I J
18. A B C D E F G H I J
19. A B C D E F G H I J
20. A B C D E F G H I J
21. A B C D E F G H I J
22. A B C D E F G H I J
23. A B C D E F G H I J
24. A B C D E F G H I J
25. A B C D E F G H I J
26. A B C D E F G H I J
27. A B C D E F G H I J
28. A B C D E F G H I J
29. A B C D E F G H I J
30. A B C D E F G H I J
31. A B C D E F G H I J
32. A B C D E F G H I J
33. A B C D E F G H I J
34. A B C D E F G H I J
35. A B C D E F G H I J
36. A B C D E F G H I J
37. A B C D E F G H I J
38. A B C D E F G H I J
39. A B C D E F G H I J
40. A B C D E F G H I J
41. A B C D E F G H I J
42. A B C D E F G H I J
43. A B C D E F G H I J
44. A B C D E F G H I J
45. A B C D E F G H I J
46. A B C D E F G H I J
47. A B C D E F G H I J
48. A B C D E F G H I J
49. A B C D E F G H I J
50. A B C D E F G H I J
51. A B C D E F G H I J
52. A B C D E F G H I J
53. A B C D E F G H I J
54. A B C D E F G H I J
55. A B C D E F G H I J
56. A B C D E F G H I J
57. A B C D E F G H I J
58. A B C D E F G H I J
59. A B C D E F G H I J
60. A B C D E F G H I J

TEST 4: Mycology and Parasitology

1. A B C D E F G H I J
2. A B C D E F G H I J
3. A B C D E F G H I J
4. A B C D E F G H I J
5. A B C D E F G H I J
6. A B C D E F G H I J
7. A B C D E F G H I J
8. A B C D E F G H I J
9. A B C D E F G H I J
10. A B C D E F G H I J
11. A B C D E F G H I J
12. A B C D E F G H I J
13. A B C D E F G H I J
14. A B C D E F G H I J
15. A B C D E F G H I J
16. A B C D E F G H I J
17. A B C D E F G H I J
18. A B C D E F G H I J
19. A B C D E F G H I J
20. A B C D E F G H I J
21. A B C D E F G H I J
22. A B C D E F G H I J
23. A B C D E F G H I J
24. A B C D E F G H I J
25. A B C D E F G H I J
26. A B C D E F G H I J
27. A B C D E F G H I J
28. A B C D E F G H I J
29. A B C D E F G H I J
30. A B C D E F G H I J
31. A B C D E F G H I J
32. A B C D E F G H I J
33. A B C D E F G H I J
34. A B C D E F G H I J
35. A B C D E F G H I J
36. A B C D E F G H I J
37. A B C D E F G H I J
38. A B C D E F G H I J
39. A B C D E F G H I J
40. A B C D E F G H I J
41. A B C D E F G H I J
42. A B C D E F G H I J
43. A B C D E F G H I J
44. A B C D E F G H I J
45. A B C D E F G H I J
46. A B C D E F G H I J
47. A B C D E F G H I J
48. A B C D E F G H I J
49. A B C D E F G H I J
50. A B C D E F G H I J

TEST 5: Infectious Diseases

1. A B C D E F G H I J
2. A B C D E F G H I J
3. A B C D E F G H I J
4. A B C D E F G H I J
5. A B C D E F G H I J
6. A B C D E F G H I J
7. A B C D E F G H I J
8. A B C D E F G H I J
9. A B C D E F G H I J
10. A B C D E F G H I J
11. A B C D E F G H I J
12. A B C D E F G H I J
13. A B C D E F G H I J
14. A B C D E F G H I J
15. A B C D E F G H I J
16. A B C D E F G H I J
17. A B C D E F G H I J
18. A B C D E F G H I J
19. A B C D E F G H I J
20. A B C D E F G H I J
21. A B C D E F G H I J
22. A B C D E F G H I J
23. A B C D E F G H I J
24. A B C D E F G H I J
25. A B C D E F G H I J
26. A B C D E F G H I J
27. A B C D E F G H I J
28. A B C D E F G H I J
29. A B C D E F G H I J
30. A B C D E F G H I J
31. A B C D E F G H I J
32. A B C D E F G H I J
33. A B C D E F G H I J
34. A B C D E F G H I J
35. A B C D E F G H I J
36. A B C D E F G H I J
37. A B C D E F G H I J
38. A B C D E F G H I J
39. A B C D E F G H I J
40. A B C D E F G H I J
41. A B C D E F G H I J
42. A B C D E F G H I J
43. A B C D E F G H I J
44. A B C D E F G H I J
45. A B C D E F G H I J
46. A B C D E F G H I J
47. A B C D E F G H I J
48. A B C D E F G H I J
49. A B C D E F G H I J
50. A B C D E F G H I J
51. A B C D E F G H I J
52. A B C D E F G H I J
53. A B C D E F G H I J
54. A B C D E F G H I J
55. A B C D E F G H I J
56. A B C D E F G H I J
57. A B C D E F G H I J
58. A B C D E F G H I J
59. A B C D E F G H I J
60. A B C D E F G H I J
61. A B C D E F G H I J
62. A B C D E F G H I J
63. A B C D E F G H I J
64. A B C D E F G H I J
65. A B C D E F G H I J
66. A B C D E F G H I J
67. A B C D E F G H I J
68. A B C D E F G H I J
69. A B C D E F G H I J
70. A B C D E F G H I J
71. A B C D E F G H I J
72. A B C D E F G H I J
73. A B C D E F G H I J
74. A B C D E F G H I J
75. A B C D E F G H I J